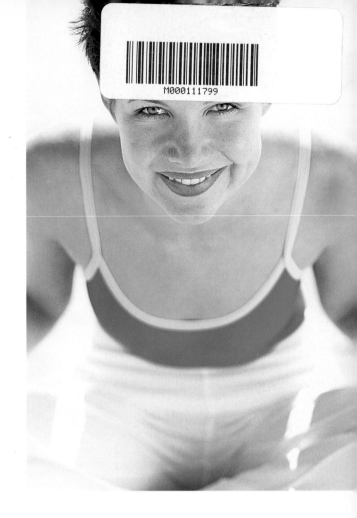

New
Again!

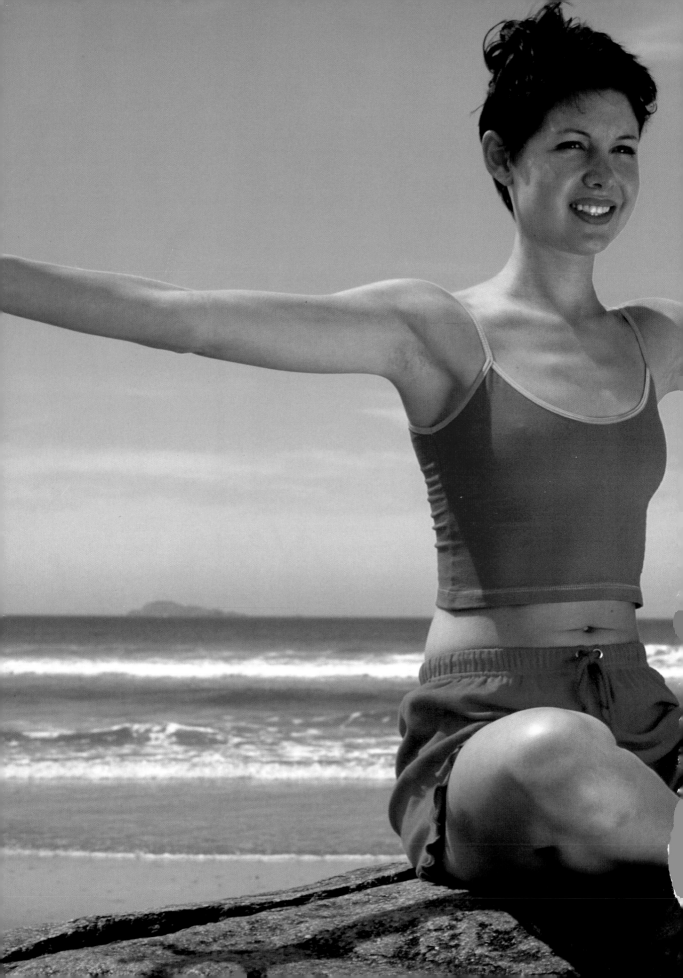

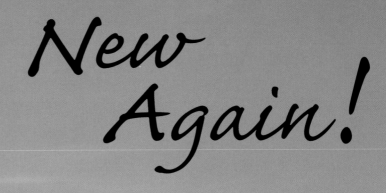

New Again!

The 28-Day Detox Plan
for Body and Soul

Anna Selby

Ulysses Press

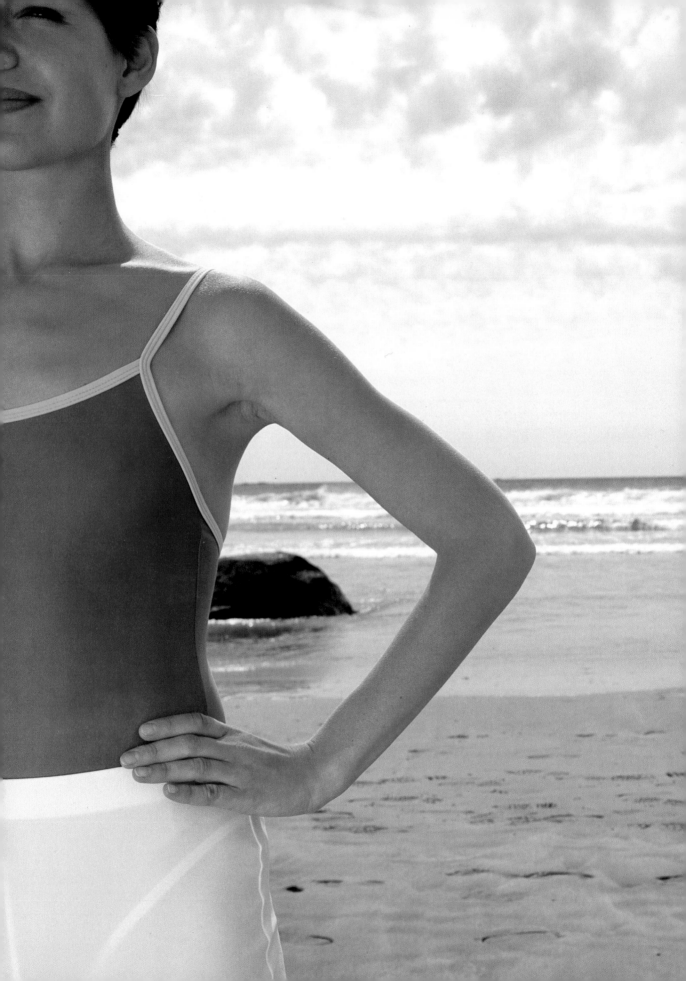

contents

6   How to use this book
8   Introduction

12   Posture
14   The roll down
16   Breathing exercise
18   Pilates
21   Stretches

28   Diet and detox
30   Why we need to detox
32   Body repair
34   The juice fast
36   Making the juices
38   More drinks
40   Juice recipes

44   Recipes
46   Breakfasts
48   Soups
52   Salads
56   Main courses

60   Exercise
62   Warm-up exercises
66   Trim torsos
70   Beautiful bottoms
76   Thigh trimmers
84   Head and shoulders above the rest!
88   Winding down
90   Aerobic exercise

92   Techniques and treatments
94   Water treatments
96   Finding relaxation
98   Meditation
104   Massage

106   One-month make-over
108   Week one
110   Week two
112   Week three
114   Week four

116   Facing the future
118   The first day of the rest of your life
120   Plan two
122   Progress charts
125   Height and weight charts

126   Index
128   Acknowledgements

Safety note

It is advisable to check with your doctor before embarking on any exercise or diet programme. The 28-Day Vitality Plan should not be considered a replacement for professional medical treatment; a physician should be consulted in all matters relating to health and particularly in respect of pregnancy and any symptoms which may require diagnosis or medical attention. While the advice and information in this book is believed to be accurate and the step-by-step instructions have been devised to avoid strain, neither the author nor the publisher can accept any legal responsibility for any injury or illness sustained while following the exercises and diet plan.

Always protect yourself from damaging sunrays. Use protective sunscreen and keep covered up when exposing yourself to the sun. Try to avoid exposure to direct sunlight during the peak radiation hours of 10am–4pm.

how to use this book

The 28-Day Vitality Plan covers almost all aspects of your daily life – what you eat and drink, how you sit and stand, the way you rest and exercise. It is designed to be used as an integrated system that progresses from week to week. For a quick overview turn to pages 106–15, which give you a week-by-week analysis of what to expect. However, before you start to get the big picture you really need to look at each section in detail to find out not only what you do on the Plan but also why you are doing it and what you can achieve from it.

The book is divided into four main sections: Posture, Diet and Detox, Exercise and Techniques and Treatments. Posture comes first for the simple reason that if you can get this right you will already look so much better and use your body so much more efficiently that you will feel a lot better about yourself. Breathing exercises come in the same section – you can't breathe properly with bad posture – and are deeply calming for the mind and bring vitality to the body at the same time.

The Diet and Detox section is crucial to the 28-Day Vitality Plan as it is centred on a prolonged detoxification designed to slough off dead and damaged (and dangerous) cells and replace them with healthy new ones. It begins with a juice fast which starts the detox off at a very deep level and, once this is finished, continues with highly nutritious foods that promote cellular renewal. You continue throughout with fresh juices, which are particularly effective at detoxing the body. The best way to get fresh juice is to make it yourself – you can buy a juicer at most department stores – because that way you drink it at its freshest and you can choose from a much greater variety of fruit and vegetables. However, you can also buy freshly squeezed juices at many supermarkets now and juice bars and some cafés also make their own. Have a look at the week-by-week section to see how the diet progresses.

The Exercise section is divided according to the body areas you want to tone. It is also very important, though, that you exercise the whole of the body, taking at least a couple of exercises from each section and building up to more difficult exercises as you progress (see the week-by-week plan). There is also an aerobic section for cardiovascular fitness and, while there are guidelines in the week-by-week plan as to how you should progress, when you start depends very much on your fitness level. If you are already a regular exerciser you naturally do not need to go back to basics, but aim to get up to the three 20-minute sessions earlier on in the programme.

Techniques and Treatments cover both mind and body. Some, like hydrotherapy and skin-brushing, aim to promote the detoxification process and stimulate the metabolism. Others, such as meditation and relaxation, calm the mind. Apart from the mental and emotional benefits of these techniques, they also have a direct physical effect – stress is itself a way of releasing toxins into the body.

The One-Month Make-Over takes you step by step through the 28-Day Vitality Plan, while Facing the Future makes a few suggestions about what to do when you've finished, as well as about how to adapt the Plan at different stages of your life. Finally, the progress charts are for you to fill in as you go along. The results will speak for themselves – by the end of the Plan you can expect to be feeling and looking 100 per cent better than when you started!

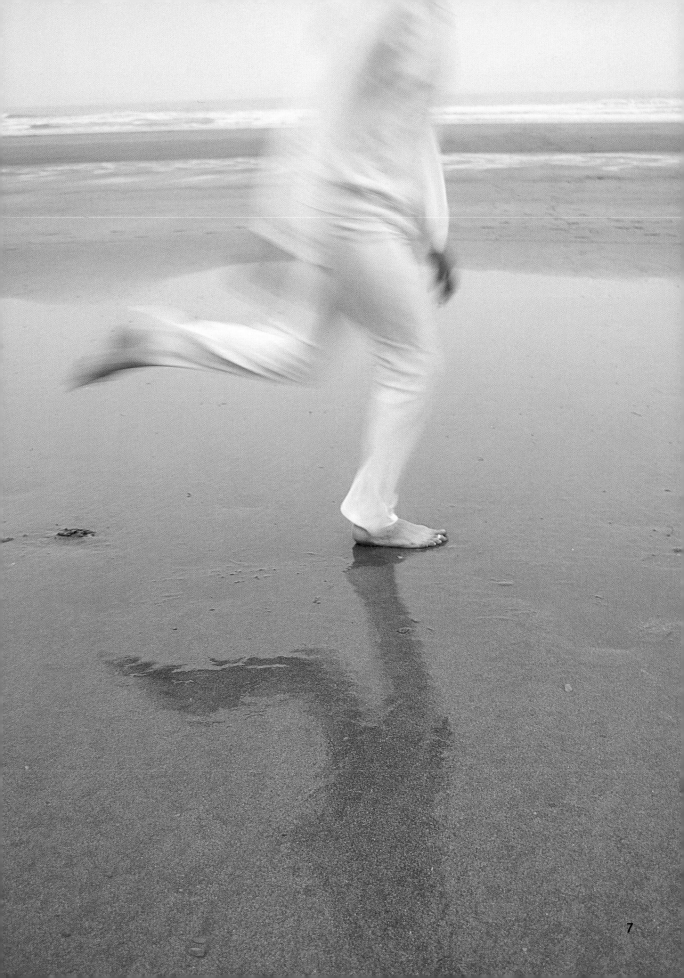

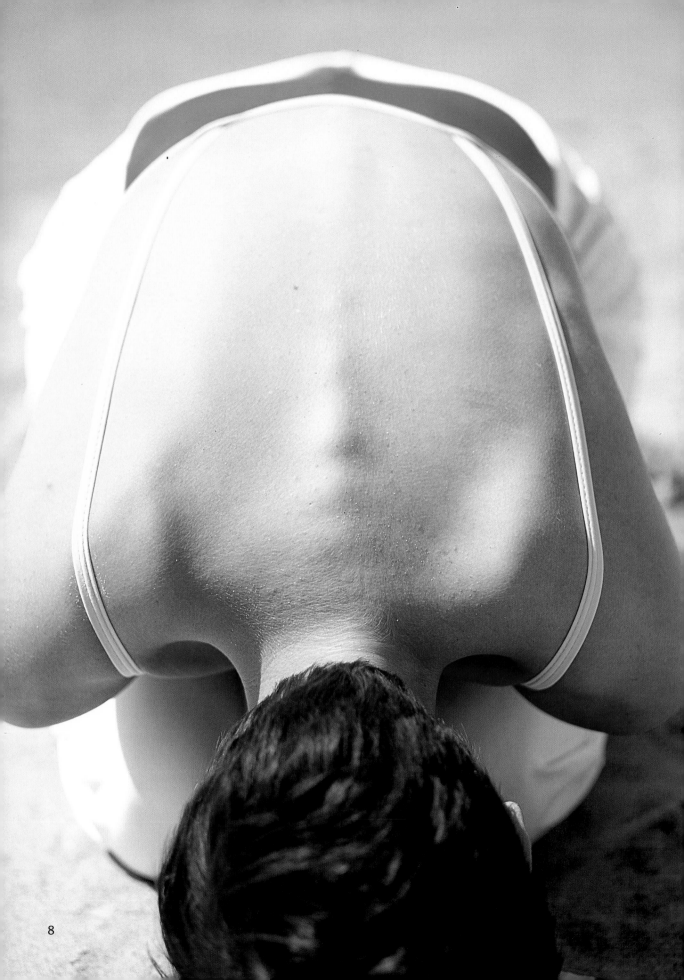

introduction

An unshapely sideways silhouette is probably what the majority of women dislike most about their bodies. We all hate those bumps and bulges and yearn for a longer, leaner shape, with a flat stomach and slimmed-down bottom and hips. It is, in fact, a perfectly achievable goal and one that can be reached in this four-week programme.

The 28-Day Vitality Plan goes further than this, though. Not only can you expect to have an improved shape, but because of the detox – the shedding of all those old, damaged or diseased cells overloading your body's ability to function – your skin and hair will look better and your energy levels will be soaring. There's no reason to hesitate – you have nothing to lose but a few unwanted pounds!

Twenty-eight days may sound like a long time to be on a diet or an exercise programme, but this is no ordinary diet. On the 28-Day Vitality Plan you do lose weight but you also lay the foundations for a better body and a healthier life where it counts – on the inside. By the end you will be looking and feeling so much better that you won't want to go back to your old bad habits, and your thinking on diet and exercise will have changed for the long term.

Many diet and exercise programmes are a chore – which is why everyone gives up halfway through. The secret of this one is that it is a pleasure. There is a delicious range of food and drinks and the exercise programme takes place on a gentle gradient – you're not expected to do strenuous exercise from the word go. On top of all that, there are plenty of delightful therapies and techniques for you to try that calm the mind and spirit while cleansing the body and making the metabolism more efficient.

All of this means that you can actually enjoy the Plan and this state of mind is in itself very important. Look at this as a special time for you. Most women spend so much time looking after other people that they never leave any time for themselves. So, while you will obviously still continue working, running a home, or looking after a family (or often nowadays all three!), you can reserve some time for yourself as well.

Another feature of the 28-Day Vitality Plan is that it gives you the chance to correct your bad habits. When you are detoxifying your system, you naturally have to stop putting more toxins in! This means that some bad habits just have to go – the worst of which is smoking, which has to stop the moment you start the Plan. Don't panic, though, if you're a smoker. It may be tough for two or three days at the beginning, but because you start with a juice fast your body feels so different so quickly it is not nearly as difficult as giving up under normal circumstances. I know this from personal experience; years ago, I used to smoke and stopped in order to do a juice fast. I felt so much better afterwards that I never went back.

Because alcohol reduces the level of vitamin absorption in the body and dehydrates it, this is also off the menu. Tea and coffee contain caffeine, which has the same effect of blocking vitamin absorption, so these are replaced with herbal teas. And any food which is not fresh and nutritious also disappears from your table – including obvious favourites like chocolate. If you want them, all of these will return at the end of the Plan – in moderation, of course!

Food intolerances

Food allergists believe a growing range of ailments can be linked to food intolerances. These are not food allergies, which have a very sudden and dramatic effect such as vomiting, a rash, anaphylactic shock or even death, though they are sometimes referred to as hidden, masked or delayed allergies. The lengthy list of food intolerance symptoms includes skin conditions such as acne, eczema and psoriasis; digestive disorders, for example colitis and irritable bowel syndrome; weight problems; hyperactivity and other behavioural problems in children; rheumatoid and osteoarthritis; insomnia, headache, migraine and exhaustion; and a range of psychological problems, such as depression.

One of the ways in which nutritionists pinpoint a food intolerance is by an elimination diet in which foods are removed from the diet and brought back gradually to monitor the effect on symptoms. During the detox, you may discover a food intolerance along the way. Because a particular food has been removed from your diet, you may discover that long-term problems, such as headache or eczema, disappear at the same time. This means you must watch very carefully for any reappearance as you return more foods to your diet. If the symptoms recur, you should be able to identify the intolerance and adapt your diet accordingly.

Positive thinking

It may seem that by putting the juice fast in the first week you start the hard way. In fact, although I have recommended three days of juice fasting as the best approach, one or two days will suffice if you find it really difficult. It is actually the first day that's the hardest so, once that is over, it does get easier! Also, you spend two days on a fruit and vegetable only diet beforehand and this prepares the body for the juice day or days to come. Many people find it much easier than they thought it was going to be. You are very likely, nevertheless, to have friends and family coaxing you to eat in case you faint or fade away. This is not going to happen, but it can be tough swimming against the tide. For this reason, it is a good idea to find a quiet time to do the juice fast part of the detox. Don't do it on working days (a long weekend is ideal) and don't make any social commitments. You want time to relax and be quiet anyway, as it often has the effect of making you want to rest more or to be tranquil and meditative. Having said that, it can also conversely give you a sudden rush of energy!

One of the reasons that the juice fast happens at the very beginning of the plan is not only that it gets the process of detoxification off to the best possible start so that the rest of the plan can build on this, but also that it has such a dramatic effect. By the end of the first week and probably before, you will be aware not just of having lost several pounds but your skin will be clearer and your hair will be softer. Quite simply, you look and feel so much better so quickly that it is the greatest possible spur to continue!

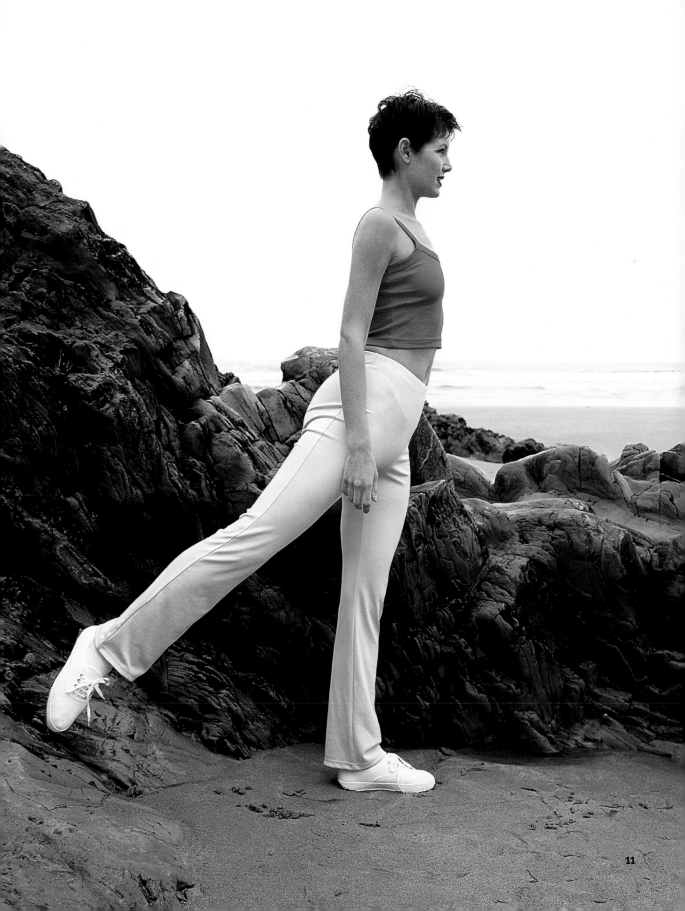

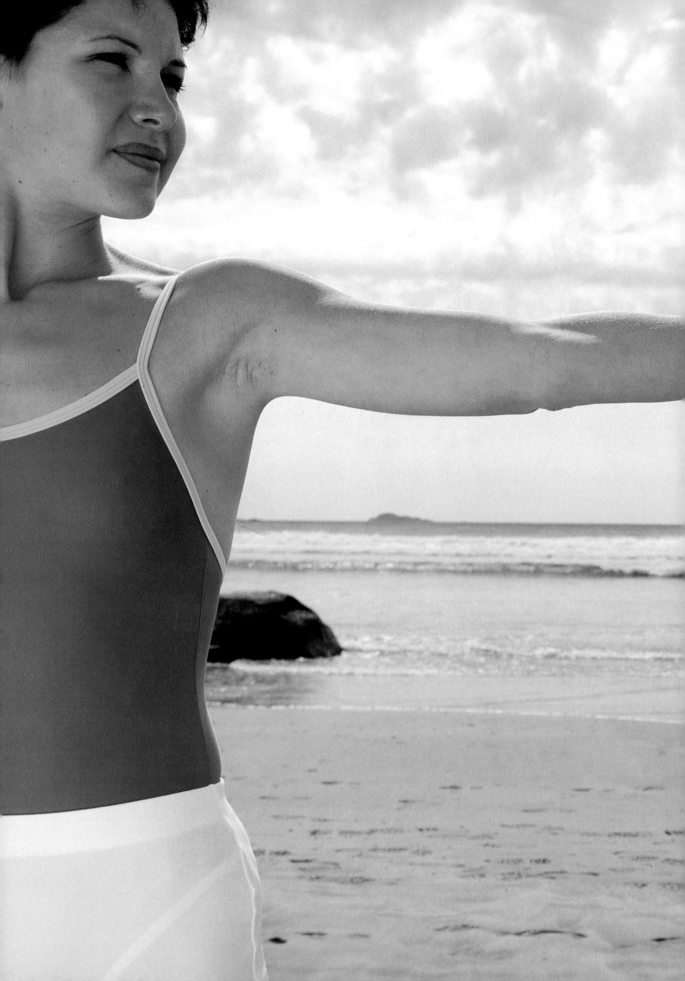

posture

Posture is an old-fashioned word, but it is of the
utmost relevance to anyone who wants to look
and feel better. If you stop slouching, you
automatically get a leaner, more pulled-up shape.
The better your posture, the more you use your
muscles even in such everyday activities as
walking around – in fact, if you exercise with bad
posture, you will not get the results you want and
you may well end up with an injury.

Good posture is really just learning to use
your body properly so that its moving parts –
arms, neck, back, legs – are in alignment. It is so
fundamental to the functioning of your body that
it also means that you are breathing properly, too.
If your shoulders are hunched or stooped or you
slouch, your internal organs do not have sufficient
room and you take less oxygen into the body,
using it less efficiently – not to mention the effect
on your digestion and circulation.

The techniques in this section – breathing
techniques, Pilates and stretching – are all aimed
towards increasing awareness of the breath and
posture and improving upon them, so that your
body is working at its peak performance when
you are exercising, as well as during the course of
your normal day.

The roll down is a deceptively simple exercise, devised to make you think about how your body connects together and then correct any postural problems. You start by putting your body into a good posture. Stand in front of a mirror and check from the top!

the roll down

Head and neck

Your neck is an integral part of your spine, so you should always keep it long and in alignment. In practical terms, this means that you should not allow your chin to jut out or tilt upwards – keep it down so that you are looking straight ahead. This position will help to release tension in the neck if you tend to store it there.

Shoulders

Like the neck, the shoulders are a common seat of tension. This means they become hunched up, and one is often higher than the other as a result of carrying a shoulder bag. Check in the mirror that your shoulders are dropped down and relaxed; if you are not sure they are in the right position or if they feel stiff or tense, do some shoulder and head circles to help you become aware of them.

Arms

You should move your arms from the centre of your back – not by lifting your shoulders. To learn how to move them, take your left arm behind your back so that the back of the hand rests on your right shoulder blade. Now slowly lift your right arm up and out from the side, feeling the movement in the back and keeping the shoulder well down. Try the same movement lifting your arm in front of you, and with your arms reversed. You will see in the mirror if you are lifting your shoulders; if they start to move, drop them back down.

Back

Backs are a common problem. Many women have S-shaped backs which make both their bottoms and their stomachs stick out. As you strengthen your stomach muscles your back will take less of the strain, so hold your stomach in and lengthen and straighten the line of your spine. Try to feel air between each vertebra. If you do this correctly, you will probably see yourself grow an inch in the mirror!

Stomach

Hold your stomach muscles lightly and firmly to take the pressure off your back. During exercise do not put too much of a strain on them, though. If they bulge out during an exercise, you are pushing them too hard too soon; build up gradually by going back to a less taxing exercise.

Legs and buttocks

Stretch out the muscles in the legs and buttocks when you are walking or exercising and try to feel them lengthening. This will improve their shape and tone.

THE ROLL DOWN

Once you have checked all the way through your posture in the mirror, the roll down will help you to feel your body in alignment.

1 Stand with your feet about 45 cm (18 inches) apart and slightly turned out, with your shoulders dropped and relaxed, your head in line with your spine and your stomach muscles held in lightly to prevent any arching in your back. Your body should feel lifted, with space between the ribs.

2 Drop your head down onto your chest and, very slowly, let the curve continue into your shoulders and back.

3 Bend your knees as you continue the curve into the waist, letting your arms drop in front of you.

4 As you bend right over, extend your arms down and rest your hands on the floor in front of you. (If you cannot reach, allow your hands to dangle – do not strain to reach the floor if this is not comfortable.) Stay there for a few seconds and let the weight of your head stretch out your spine. Now, very slowly, roll the body back up. Feel your buttock muscles working to anchor the base of your spine and keep your stomach held in. As your knees straighten again, your legs lengthen and your back places itself vertebra by vertebra into a tall, elongated position. Your head comes up last, in line with your spine. Do this exercise several times so that you can really feel the placement of your body. Always start with a roll down before you exercise – and it's a good way to wake up your body in the morning, too.

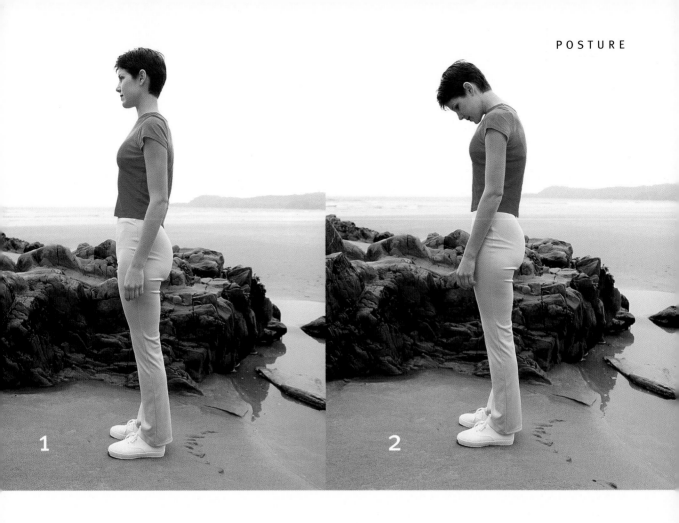

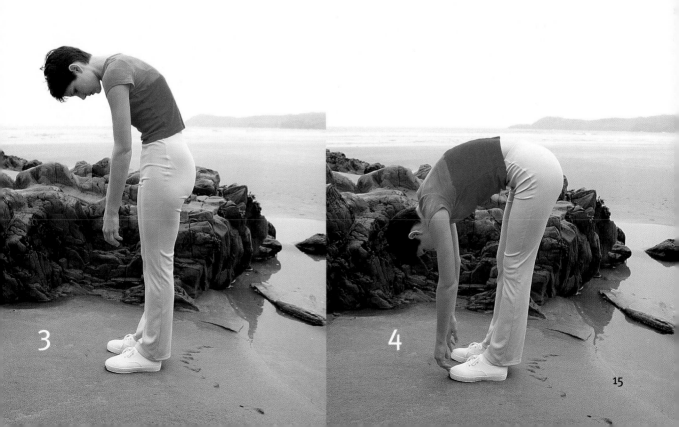

1

2

3

4

breathing exercise

Breathing is something we do automatically – we simply don't think about it. Of course, it would be very difficult to think about our breathing all the time, but it is useful to spend a few minutes each day doing full, healthy breathing because most of us breathe so shallowly, using only the upper chest and about a third of our lung capacity, that only a small proportion of the oxygen that should be reaching our bloodstream is inhaled. As the lungs fail to fill properly over the years, they lose their elasticity and so cannot reach full capacity.

This poor breathing may be merely a habit and is often related to stress. The more tense we feel, the shallower our breathing is likely to become. And, just as tension and shallow breathing often bring with them thoughts galloping out of control, slow, deep breathing calms the mind. The breathing routine here is designed to be used on a regular, preferably twice-daily basis, morning and evening, but it can also come in handy when you're in a stressful situation – you don't have to lie down.

Breathing and exercise

One of the great benefits of aerobic exercise is that it improves the way we use oxygen. However, we often do not breathe correctly when we exercise and this undoes all the benefits. Most of us tend to hold our breath whenever we do anything strenuous, but this actually makes whatever we are doing more difficult and encourages the accumulation of tensions in the body. By breathing correctly during exercise, we can actually rid the body of those tensions.

Rather than holding the breath or gasping it in, breathe out as you make an effort and in as you release it. This helps you to perform any exercise better, aids concentration and revitalizes your energy levels. This way of breathing will help a great deal in the exercises on the following pages – so try to keep a careful watch on your breathing as you do them.

BREATHING ROUTINE

1 Lie down flat on your back, either on the floor or on a bed. You can put a thin cushion under your neck or your lower back if you feel you need support. Place one hand on your ribcage and the other on your abdomen.

2 Inhale on a slow count of 5 and try to feel the oxygen pouring into your lungs all the way down into your abdomen. Feel first your abdomen rise and then your ribs extend outwards so that your hands move.

Hold the breath at its fullest point for another slow count of 5.

Now let the breath out on another slow count of 5 through the mouth. As you do so, feel the abdomen and then the ribs return to their normal positions.

Rest for a few moments and then repeat, continuing for around 5 minutes.

1

2

pilates

The Pilates system originated in Germany around 90 years ago, when a frail child called Joseph Pilates took up body building to increase his strength. The programme he devised was so successful that by the age of 14 he was posing for anatomical drawings. He called his system 'muscle contrology', its aim being to bring about the complete co-ordination of the body, mind and spirit working with – not on, or against – the body's muscles. In 1924, Pilates and his wife Clara moved to New York, where he opened his now world-famous studio. Dancers were the first to flock there – George Balanchine, Martha Graham, Jerome Robbins, Ruth St Denis – and sportsmen, actors and the public followed.

A Pilates studio uses some rather curious-looking pieces of equipment, with springs, pulleys, bars, handles and weights. They all tone and firm the body, and are designed to produce a beautiful, effortless posture with stomach and bottom pulled in, tension-free shoulders and the merest hollow in your back rather than a huge sway. These are gentle exercises that help release tension and stretch out the body into a graceful shape. The exercises shown here are typical of the Pilates system but can be done without special equipment.

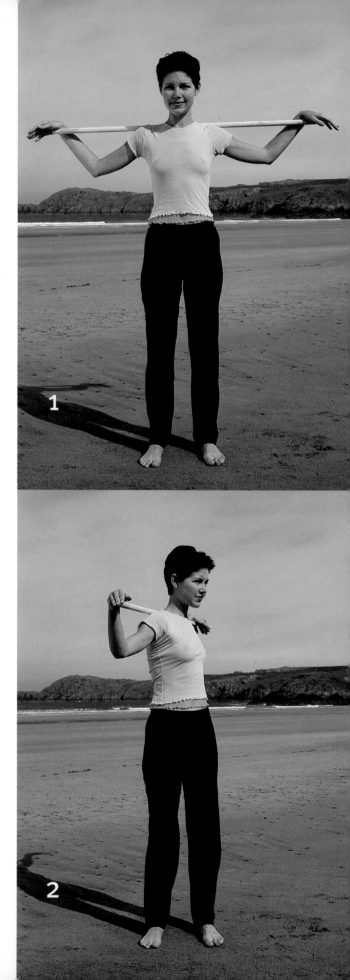

WAIST TWISTS

You need a broom handle for this exercise, which not only works on the waist but also opens up the shoulder area.

1 Stand with your feet hip-width apart and the pole across your shoulders, the hands resting on the ends. Feel your spine long and your neck and head lifted.

2 As you breathe out, twist your body slowly as far as you can without letting your hips move. Repeat for 8 turns on each side.

SINGLE LEG STRETCHES

1 Lie flat on the floor, your body lengthened, your stomach pushing back towards your spine and your upper body relaxed. Place your legs together, with your feet pointed. Draw your knees up to your chest and curve your head and shoulders up from the floor. Rest your hands on your legs, just behind your knees.

2 Stretch out one leg, keeping it close to the floor and pointing your toes, meanwhile gently pulling the bent leg closer towards your chest.

3 Draw the extended leg back in and stretch out the other leg, again holding the bent leg against the chest. Repeat, alternating 16 times, making sure to stretch the extended leg as far as possible each time.

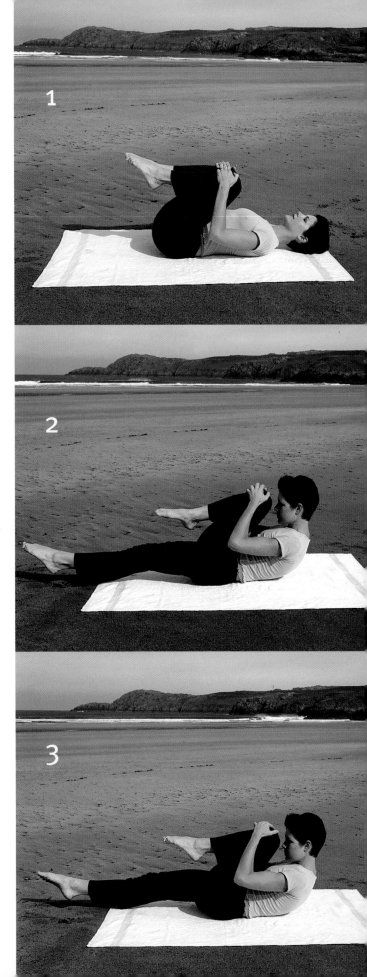

THE CAT

This cat-like stretch should not be attempted if you have any weakness in the back.

1 Position yourself on all fours, knees in line with your hips, arms in line with your shoulders, fingers facing forwards. Your head should be in one long line from your spine and your spine should be absolutely straight.

2 Breathing out, pull in your stomach and form as high and open an arch with your back as you can.

3 Breathe in as you return to the starting position then, as you breathe out, drop your back and lift your head so that you are looking upwards. Repeat the whole sequence slowly 4 times. If you have any concerns about the strength of your back, miss out the second part of the exercise.

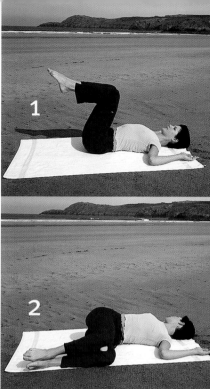

TENNIS BALL

1 Lie on your back, your arms out from the shoulders, elbows bent. Bend your knees and raise your legs so that your thighs are at right angles to your body.

2 Place a tennis ball between your knees. (You can do this exercise without the tennis ball, but it does help you to keep your knees firmly together.) Keeping your thighs at right angles to your body, breathe out and let your knees drop down to your left towards the floor while your head turns to the right. Breathe in and feel the diagonal stretch then, as you breathe out, lift your knees back up to the centre and take them down to the other side, again with your head turning in the opposite direction. Repeat 8 times in each direction.

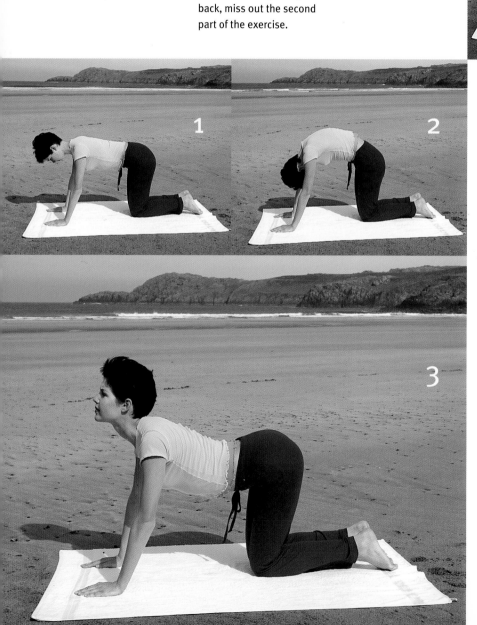

stretches

Stretches not only elongate the body, they are also very relaxing. For the best results do them after you have exercised, when the muscles are well warmed up. They are excellent at releasing tension stored in the body, and the end result will be particularly good if you follow them with a deep relaxation technique (see pages 96–7).

BACK STRETCH

Tension is often held in the back, either along the spine or in the shoulders or neck. This stretch helps to iron out the knots.

Stand with your legs hip-width apart and hold on to the back of a chair or a table with your fingertips just able to reach it. Lengthen your spine as far as you can, with your head dropped to release any tensions in the neck or shoulders. Hold the stretch for at least 1 minute, breathing deeply, and you will feel the spine extend further.

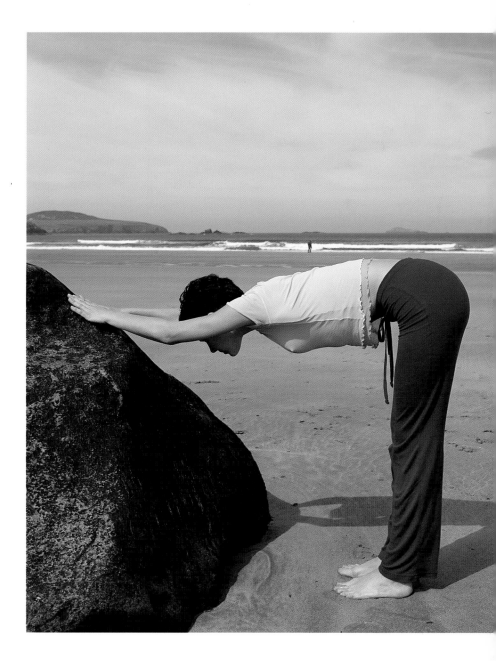

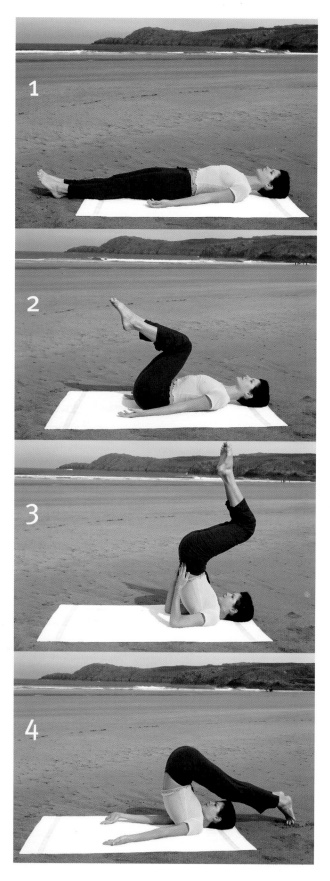

THE PLOUGH

1 Lie flat on the floor, legs together, arms slightly out from your sides and hands palm upwards.

2 Breathe in and bend your knees into your chest, keeping your neck long.

3 As you breathe out, start to raise your back from the floor, supporting your hips with your hands.

4 Keep on rolling up so that your feet are pointing behind your head. Keeping your back straight, take your legs over your head and drop your feet down towards or onto the floor behind – the more supple and stretched your back becomes, the further your feet will go. When you are comfortable in this position, you can flex the feet back so they are 'on the walk' with the toes curled under. This will increase the stretch. To come out of the pose, raise your legs, drop your knees down to your chest and roll the spine down slowly, finally stretching out your legs on the floor.

THE SHOULDER STAND

1, 2 & 3 Begin as for the plough but this time, instead of sending your legs behind you, lift them upwards, straightening out your spine until you reach a vertical position. This takes a fair amount of practice! When your legs are raised and your feet pointed, press your chin onto your chest. This stimulates the thyroid and parathyroid glands, which is suggested delays ageing. Close your eyes, breathe deeply and try to relax into the position.

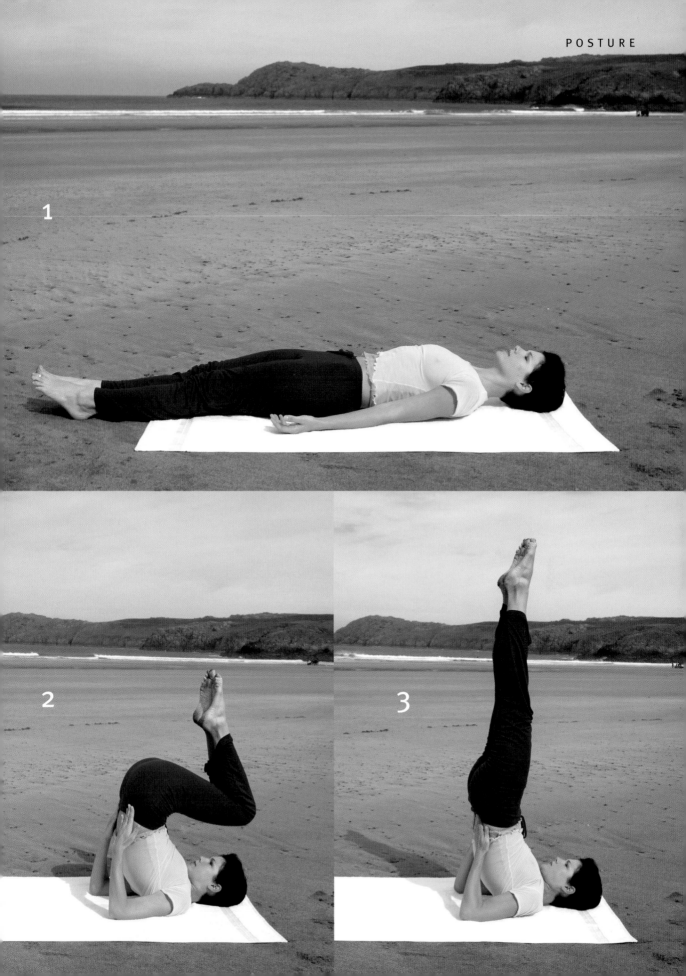

1

2

3

SALUTE TO THE SUN

This is one of the best-known – and best – yoga *asanas*. It stretches your whole body, as well as giving an internal massage to various organs.

1 Stand very tall with your stomach held in, your buttocks tucked under and your back straight. Hold your hands together in a prayer position just in front of your breastbone. Breathe in deeply and then exhale.

2 & 3 Breathe in deeply and stretch your arms over your head. Stretching your arms further back, lean back and drop your head back. Return to a upright position.

4 & 5 Breathing out, bend forward from the hips with a straight back. Dropping your head and stretching your back right down, try to get your hands to the floor.
If you cannot, try to hold the backs of your ankles but don't force this if it is hard to do.

6 Breathe in, bend your left leg and, resting your hands on the floor, take your right leg out behind you, stretching it fully. Look upwards.

7 Take your left leg back so that it is in line with the right and you are supported on your arms. Hold this position for a moment and then raise your hips so that your body forms a triangle with the floor, with your head dropped. Breathe out.

8 Supporting your weight on your hands, drop your knees and chest to the ground, with your hips still held as high as you can.

9 Breathe in, drop your hips to the ground and then, breathing out, arch your upper body back and look upwards.

10 Breathe out and lift back up to the triangle shape, stretching out and trying to press your heels down into the floor.

11 Breathe in and bring your right leg forward, knee to your chest, stretching your left leg out behind you. Look up as you breathe out.

12 Breathe in and, as you breathe out, take your left leg forward to meet your right and begin to straighten your legs. Keep your back straight and aim to press your body against your legs, with your head remaining dropped towards the ground. Bend your knees, if you need to. If you are very flexible, for extra stretch you can pull your body closer by clasping the backs of your ankles.

13 Breathe in, raising your body from the hips and bending back to look upwards with an arched back and arms outstretched.

14 Breathe out and return to the starting prayer position. Repeat up to 10 times. With 10 repeats, Salute to the Sun is virtually a work-out on its own.

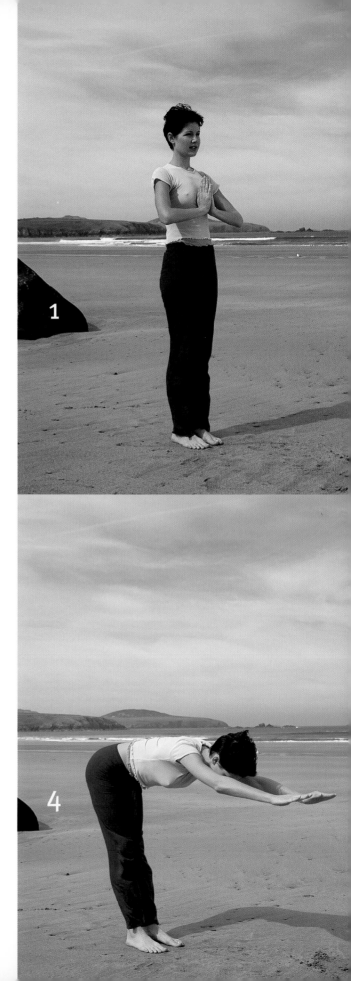

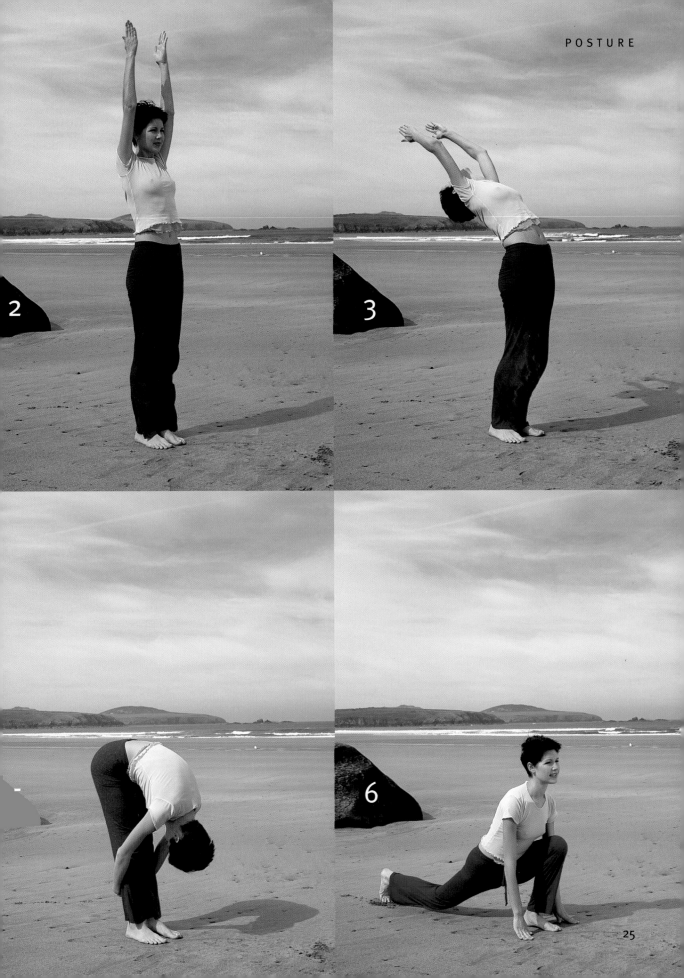

2

3

6

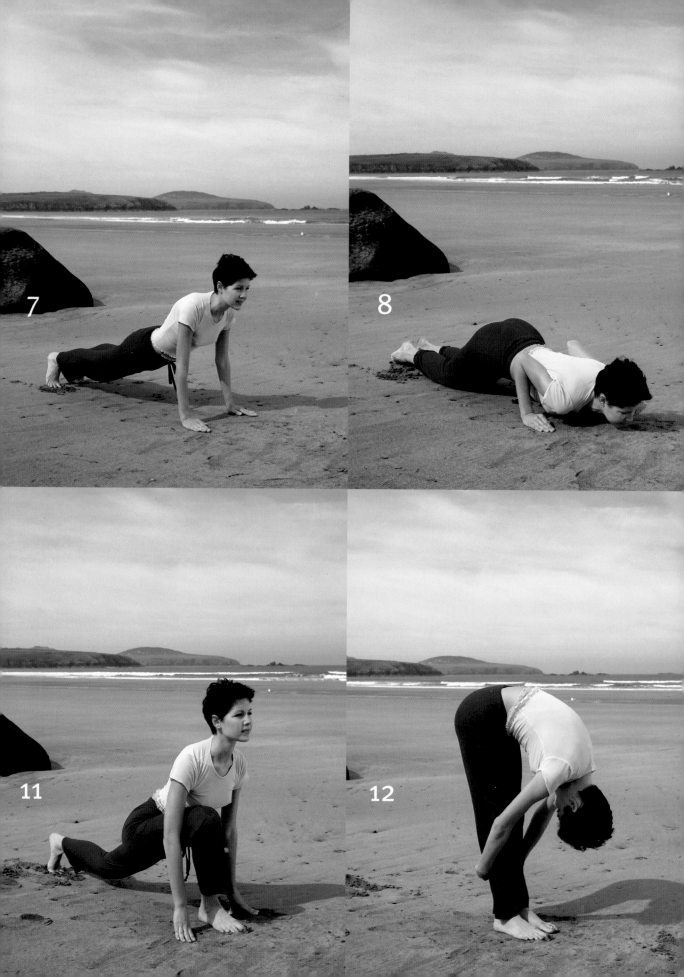

9

10

13

14

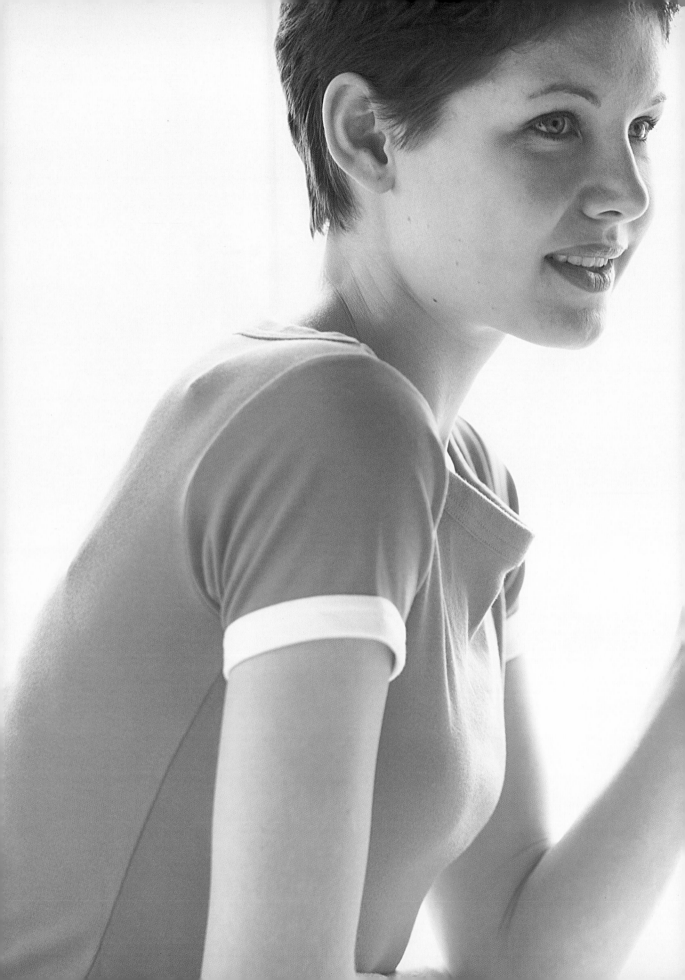

diet
and detox

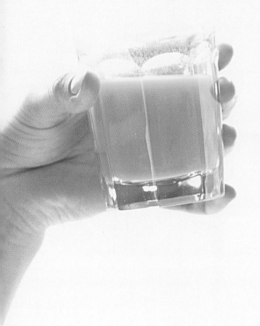

Twentieth-century living is a dangerous business. Our bodies are under constant assault from pollution, stress, bad posture, sedentary jobs and our own bad eating habits. Over the months and years, the effects build up and emerge in many different forms – everything from passing infections, skin eruptions, headaches and digestive problems to serious conditions, such as ulcers, cancer and heart disease.

The more we overload our bodies, the further they sink under the strain. When we detox, we do the opposite – we give our bodies the chance to repair and cleanse and restore a more balanced state to the entire system. And it shows. As well as losing any excess weight, you can expect to have clear skin, healthy-looking hair, strong nails and more energy. Detox also has a very calming effect on the mind, particularly if you combine it with one of the relaxation techniques or meditation (see pages 96–103). And, most importantly of all, it sets you on the right course for your long-term health. Once you've done the 28-Day Vitality Plan, you'll want to stay feeling this good.

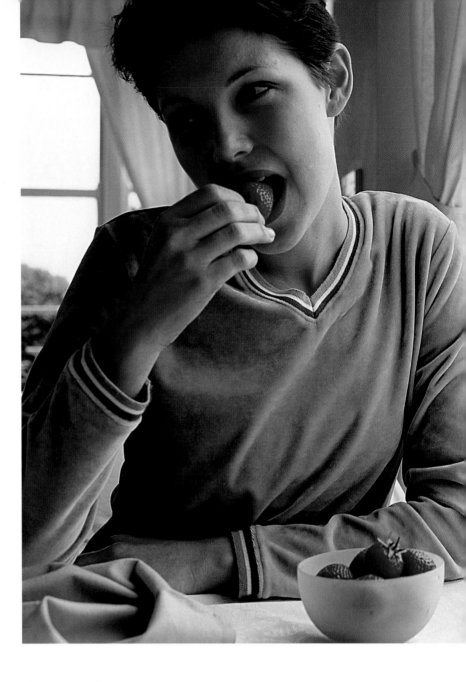

why we need to detox

These days, we all live at a pace that would have seemed unbelievable, and indeed impossible, to our grandparents. We have demanding jobs – and often have to travel long distances to get to them – we keep later and longer hours, we run homes, bring up children and usually try to fit in hectic social lives, too. It's no surprise then that we become tired and run down, never feeling on top of things. And because time is the one thing most of us don't have enough of, we cut corners. We eat convenience or junk food, we don't get enough sleep, we can't fit in exercise and we often drink too much or smoke as a quick-fix way to

relax. Deep down, we all know this is no way to live, but we may not be aware of the very real dangers this lifestyle presents.

Body renewal

Our bodies are extremely complex organisms in a state of constant growth and renewal on a cellular level. They get rid of old, damaged and dead cells and replace them with new ones on a daily basis. There is also a system of priorities for the metabolism – for instance, if we fall ill, our body concentrates its energies on repelling invading infections and the healing

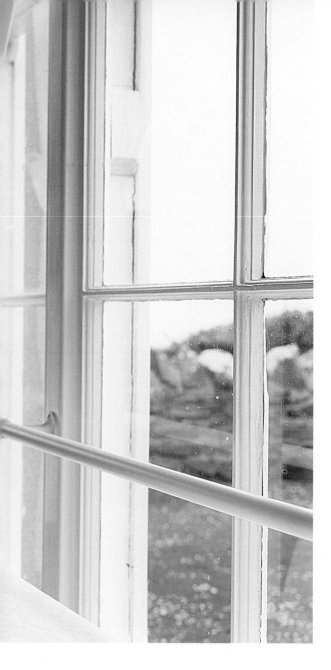

elimination of old toxins and promote cell renewal. And, as you rejuvenate the cells, you become healthier and you look and feel younger! A tall order from just a change of diet? Far from it. It is universally accepted that high-fat, processed, salty foods are linked to heart disease and many other serious conditions have also been linked to diet; the World Health Organization has found that around 85 per cent of adult cancers are avoidable and of these around half are related to dietary deficiencies. It isn't that we don't eat enough – most people in the developed world eat too much. But the food we're eating has lost much of its nutritional value through processing and is packed full of fat, sugar and nutritionally worthless preservatives, colourings and flavourings instead.

Super scavengers

In particular, the World Health Organization has said that vitamins A (beta-carotene from vegetable sources), C and E are vital for health. These vitamins, together with the mineral selenium, are known as anti-oxidants. They can protect us not only against minor infections but also serious degenerative diseases such as cancer and heart disease, as well as conditions that come with premature ageing. They work by acting as scavengers for free radicals. Free radicals are electrochemically unbalanced molecules, generated within our bodies by, among other things, pollution, cigarettes, pesticides, drugs, certain foods, overeating and stress. Free radical molecules are responsible, on a cellular level, for many of the things that go wrong with the body. They react with other, healthy molecules to make them unstable, too, and a chain reaction can start up, which leads to a process of cellular destruction and disease.

We clearly need as many anti-oxidants as we can get! One of the best places to find them is in fresh fruit and vegetables and that is why these foods are vital for detoxing. Many nutrients, however, are destroyed by cooking and that is why raw food is so much more effective as a source of health – and so is at the core of the 28-Day Vitality Plan.

process. When we pour toxins into our bodies, too, it treats these as a matter of urgency and works on processing them to render them harmless. What this means, though, is that there is less energy for the everyday processes of cleansing, healing and renewal. Over time, the body can't keep up the pace, the strain shows on the overworked liver and kidneys and the body's performance slows down.

When we detox, two things happen. First, we stop overloading the body with harmful substances and, secondly, we give it plenty of the right nutrients to actually speed up the

body repair

Your body knows how to cleanse and restore itself – during detoxification, you are simply giving it a helping hand. For the deepest and swiftest detoxification, you should not only stop adding new toxins but help it in the cleansing process. The liver and kidneys, the main organs of detoxification, will do most of the work: the liver renders harmless the toxins that enter our body or eliminates them altogether, while the kidneys filter out toxins in the blood and eliminate them in the urine.

How the detox works

During the 28-Day Vitality Plan, the daily workload of new toxins to be processed is lifted, giving these important organs the opportunity to work on the store of old ones. There is time to cleanse and repair long-standing damage and the body starts straight away. It rids itself of tissues that are diseased, damaged or dead, and as these are eliminated the building up of new healthy cells speeds up.

The first week of the Plan consists of raw food only with, at its core, a juice fast. Raw food and fresh juices have a remarkably cleansing and regenerating effect on the entire system as they retain all of their nutrients, which can be destroyed in processing and cooking. Low in calories and high in fibre, they are packed with anti-oxidants to accelerate healing and are particularly effective at cleansing the gut. Juices are an essential part of the process. They are very easily assimilated by the body and contain all the nutrients present in raw fruit and vegetables. And, because it's easier to drink juice than it is to eat huge quantities of raw vegetables or fruit, you can obtain a lot more fresh, natural nutrients than in any other way.

After the juice fast, you gradually return to a normal diet but with the emphasis still on raw food and juices, so the detoxification process continues. In the second and third weeks there is a wide range of delicious soups and salads to choose from. And, in the fourth week, you establish a healthy diet for the future.

The first week may look a bit daunting, but don't be put off – it's actually much easier than you think. You will need, though, to find a time when you are not going to be very busy or stressed or having a particularly social time – with all the temptations of food and drink that go with it! Try to fit the juice fast itself into a long weekend when you can find some quiet time on your own or with a friend who wants to do it with you.

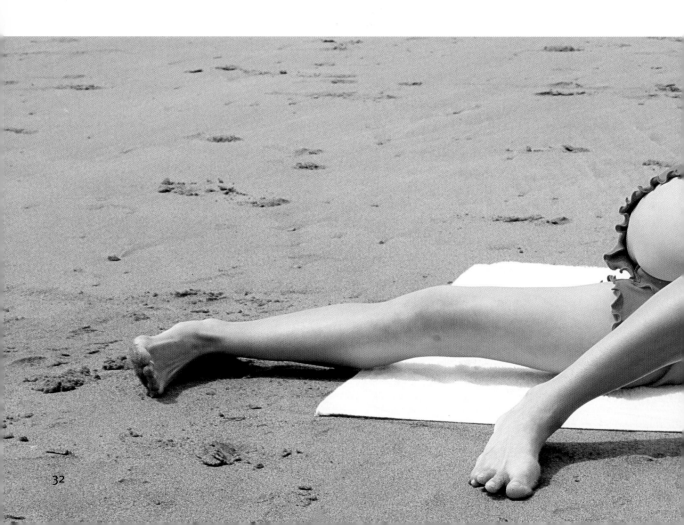

Now, take a deep breath because there are some things that you have to cut out for the next 28 days so that the detoxification process can work. They are:

- Smoking

- Alcohol – it reduces the level of vitamin absorption in the body, as well as causing dehydration

- Any food that is not part of the plan

- Over-the-counter drugs – but check with your doctor about prescribed drugs

- Tea and coffee – these both contain caffeine which, far from being a nutrient, interferes with the absorption of vitamins. It is also addictive.

After the first few days, when you may well have withdrawal symptoms, you'll find you feel better, look better and have much more energy. It really is worth it!

The rules of fasting

Many people get very worried about the idea of fasting; they think that if you miss a meal, you'll faint or fade away. Nothing could be further from the truth. You will actually end up with more energy, not less. I have worked out the detox on the basis of a three-day juice fast, but if you find this daunting try it for one or two days instead. You may even find you want to continue for the full three once you begin – and bear in mind that it is the first day that is the hardest.

There are some people who should not fast. They include: women who are pregnant or breastfeeding, children, the frail and elderly, anyone with diabetes, TB, advanced heart disease, kidney dysfunction, or any degenerative disease, and anyone who is underweight. Everyone should, in any case, have a check-up with their doctor first.

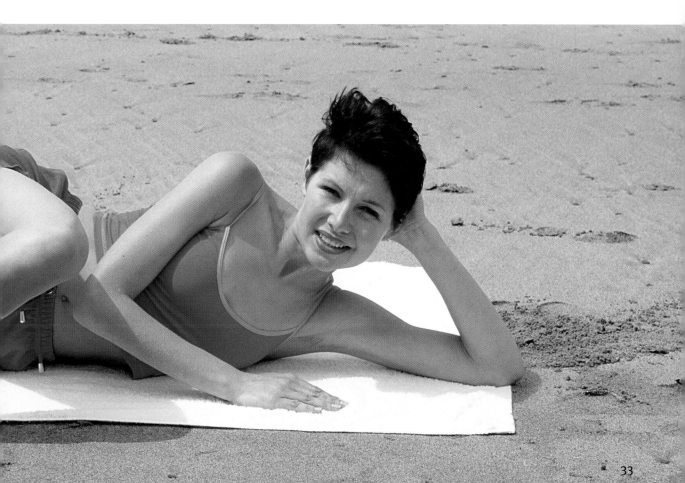

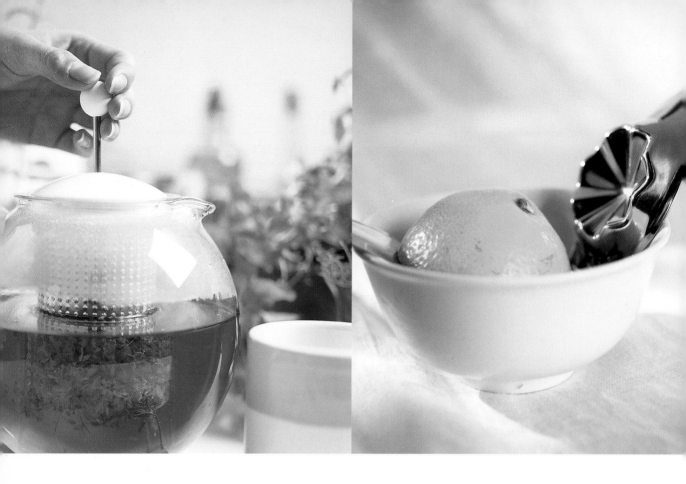

the juice fast

The juice fast can last between one and three days. Obviously, the detoxing effects of three days will be greater than for one, but if you decide to do only a one-day fast, have an extra day of preparation and an extra day of the fast-breaking. If you do a two-day fast, have an extra day of preparation. The preparation for the fast is very important; it starts the cleansing process and minimizes side-effects. Breaking the fast is equally important – you have to come back to food slowly or you'll overload the digestive system, undo all you've achieved and even feel quite unwell.

I've put the juice fast at the start of the programme because apart from the immediate internal cleansing effects it does have such a visible effect, too. You will see weight loss and an improvement in your skin, hair and nails. By the end of the week you will have more energy, and as you already look and feel so much better you won't find it hard to keep to the rest of the programme.

Side-effects

Having said that, as soon as your body starts to clear itself of toxins, some side-effects are inevitable as the toxins make their way out. These are nothing to worry about – in fact, they are a sign that the detox is working. The following common side-effects are only temporary and they will be replaced by a feeling of general well-being by the end of the week.

Furry tongue This happens to everyone. Clean your teeth frequently and scrape your tongue with the toothbrush a few times.

Headache This is very common if there was a lot of caffeine, chocolate, alcohol or sugar in your diet. Don't take any medication. Drink extra fluids, rest and dab some lavender oil onto your temples.

Irritability Try to expose yourself to as little outside stress as possible. Do some relaxation or meditation. Exercise often helps and so, if the irritability stems from tiredness, does rest.

Excessive elimination Great! It's not really excessive even if you find you need to urinate every half hour at times. This is just the toxins coming out and is particularly likely if you've had water retention. Loose bowels are also possible as with any change of diet and so, paradoxically, is constipation. These problems usually normalize within a few days.

Flu and cold symptoms Runny nose and eyes, aches and pains are all quite common and only temporary.

Skin eruptions Many toxins are eliminated through the skin, so you may get spots on the face or body. Baths or showers once or twice daily are important to wash the toxins away. The skin will clear by the end of the week, by which time it is usually glowing with health.

Tiredness Some people do feel tired, particularly if they've been under a lot of stress. Rest if you need to – higher energy levels will replace the tiredness soon.

The first two days

These are very important to prepare the body. Make sure you get plenty of rest.

Breakfast Natural yogurt with seeds. Apple and carrot juice.

Mid-morning Apple.

Lunch As much salad as you like made from any of the following raw ingredients: bean sprouts, beetroot, broccoli, carrots, celery, chicory, cucumber, peppers, radishes, spring onions, watercress and any kind of salad leaves. Dress with a little yogurt and black pepper. Any vegetable juice from pages 42–3.

Mid-afternoon Apple.

Supper As much fruit salad as you like, made with fresh fruit and a little orange or apple juice to sweeten. Again, you can have a couple of spoonfuls of natural yogurt with this. Choose a fruit juice from pages 40–1.

Drink plenty of herb teas and water throughout the day – aim for around 1.8 litres (3 pints) at least.

The juice fast

7 am	Start the day with the juice of a lemon squeezed into hot water.
8 am	Herb tea or water.
9 am	Apple and carrot juice.
10.30 am	Herb tea or water.
12 am	Vegetable broth (see page 38).
2 pm	Herb tea or water.
3.30 pm	Fruit juice (choose from pages 40–1).
5 pm	Herb tea or water.
6.30 pm	Vegetable broth (see page 38).
8 pm	Vegetable juice (choose from pages 42–3).
9.30 pm	Herb tea or water.

Breaking the fast

Coming off the fast is as important as the fast itself, so follow this plan carefully.

Day One

7 am	Juice of a lemon squeezed into hot water.
8 am	Herb tea or water.
9 am	One apple.
11 am	Carrot and apple juice.
1 pm	Vegetable broth, bowl of immune-boosting soup (see page 50).
2.30 pm	Herb tea or water.
4 pm	Vegetable juice.
5.30 pm	Herb tea or water.
7 pm	Vegetable broth.
8.30 pm	Fruit juice.
9.30 pm	Herb tea or water.

Day Two

7 am	Juice of a lemon squeezed into hot water.
8 am	Herb tea or water.
9 am	A small bowl of prunes soaked in juice overnight.
10.30 am	Carrot and apple juice.
12 am	Vegetable broth and a small bowl of fresh vegetable salad, dressed with a squeeze of lemon and pepper.
2 pm	Herb tea or water.
3.30 pm	Fruit juice with an apple.
5 pm	Bowl of immune-boosting soup.
6.30 pm	Herb tea or water.
8 pm	Vegetable juice and vegetable broth.
9.30 pm	Herb tea or water.

Day Three

7 am	Juice of a lemon squeezed into hot water.
8 am	Herb tea or water.
9 am	Small bowl of soaked prunes with 3 tablespoons live natural yogurt.
10.30 am	Carrot and apple juice.
12 am	Vegetable broth, vegetable salad as Day Two with a baked potato, dressed with live natural yogurt.
2.30 pm	Herb tea or water.
4 pm	Fruit juice with an apple.
5.30 pm	Herb tea or water.
7 pm	Vegetable broth, immune-boosting soup with a slice of wholemeal bread.
8 pm	Vegetable juice.
9.30 pm	Herb tea or water.

making the juices

Although there are plenty of juices on the supermarket shelves, they bear little resemblance to those you make with a juicer either in taste or in nutritional value. There are a few freshly squeezed juices available to buy (usually orange, apple and carrot) and you can make do with these if you don't want to spend money on a juicer. However, once you've tasted real juice, you'll want to keep on making it long after you've finished the 28-Day Vitality Plan.

Preparing the fruits and vegetables

When you make juice, try to get organic fruit and vegetables if you can as these will not have been treated with chemical fertilizers, pesticides or herbicides. Choose fruit that is ripe, as it will be easier both to juice and to digest. Don't buy any produce that is bruised or obviously past its best. All fruit and vegeta-

bles need to be very thoroughly cleaned because you use them whole – many nutrients are just below the surface of the skin. Leaves, tops and outer skins and peel on vegetables such as carrots, celery, beetroot and root vegetables all go in. Juice all the leaves – even the less appetizing outer ones on green leafy vegetables. Some fruits such as bananas and citrus fruits (though generally the latter are not recommended for a fast) need to be peeled, but many don't; a strong juicing machine can cope with the skins of papaya, mango and any kind of melon, for example. Large stones, such as those of cherries, plums, mangos, apricots or peaches, should be removed but the smaller pips of apples and grapes can be juiced, too.

Home-made juices do not look the same as those out of a carton. They may be a rather murky-looking colour and they may also have a much thicker consistency, sometimes with a

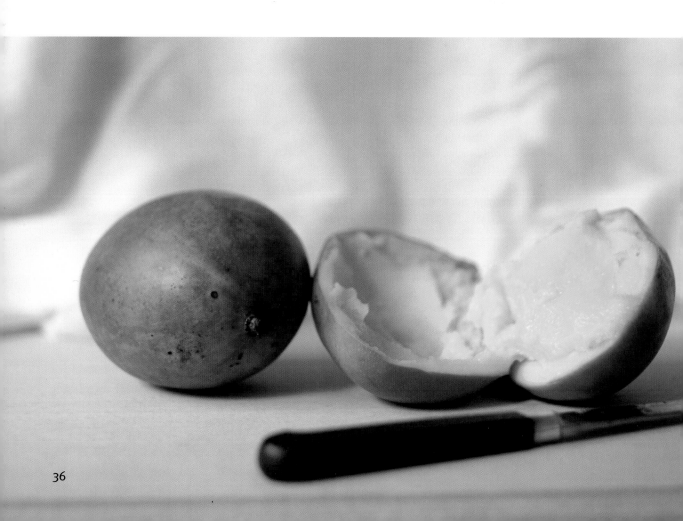

froth on top, and a much more powerful taste. You don't need to strain the juice, even if it does have a froth – give it a stir and drink it as soon as you've made it.

Buying a juicer

You can't make juice with a blender or food processor unless there is a separate juicing attachment. This is because they will make a purée of the whole fruit or vegetable, while a juicer separates the fibrous pulp from the juice. Juicers are now very affordable – they start at around £30 – but they can also go up to more than £200! Besides the price, there is also the question of how trouble-free the juicer is to use. This is mainly down to how easy it is to clean – the pulps and fibres can get lodged in awkward corners so it's very important to get a machine that you can take apart and put together again without fuss, with all its parts accessible.

Types of juicers

There are a number of types of juicers that carry out the job in different ways.

Centrifugal juicers Vegetables and fruits are grated into tiny pieces and spun around at high speed with the liquid being extracted by centrifugal force – hence the name. The juice pours into a jug, while the fibrous pulp is left behind. Centrifugal juicers tend to be the lowest in price. You need to add the fruit and vegetables gradually so they don't block up. If you're juicing something very fibrous, an apple or carrot will help keep the machine clear.

Triturating juicers These tear up the vegetables and fruit and force the pulp against a screen with the pressure of a rotating cutter. They are slower than centrifugal juicers, but because they do not whip the contents around – which means more oxidization because of a prolonged exposure to the air – triturators are held to make juice that has a somewhat higher nutritional content. They are more expensive than centrifugal juicers and also tend to take up more room in the kitchen.

Hydraulic juice presses Presses use immense force to squeeze the juice out of fruits and vegetables. The juice comes out through a filter into a jug and has more nutrients than that from any other type of juicer. These machines are, however, the most expensive.

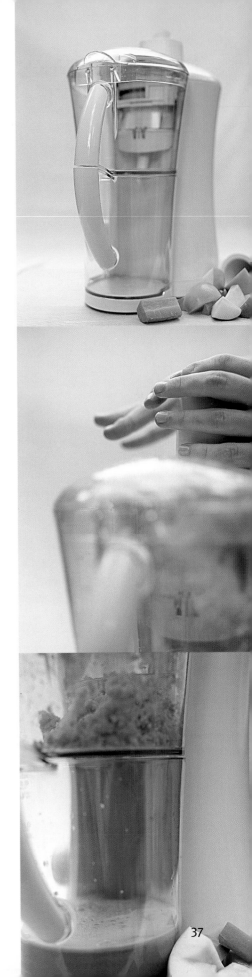

more drinks

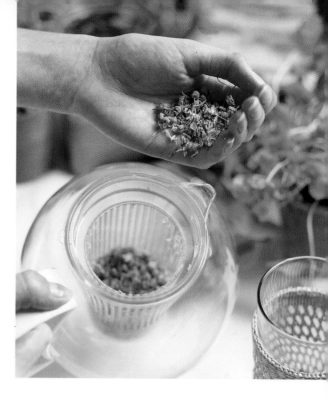

Besides the juices, there are several other important drinks that you take during the course of the 28-Day Vitality Plan.

Vegetable broth

This should be freshly made each day. It makes a cleansing and alkalizing hot drink, supplying vitamins, minerals and trace elements. As with the juices, organic is best, but if organic vegetables are not available make sure you clean the produce particularly well.

2 large potatoes
2 carrots
4 celery sticks, including leaves
2 beetroot (uncooked), including leaves
at least two other vegetables including one green one, such as cabbage, turnips, spinach, spring greens, parsnips, sweet potatoes, leeks, onions
flavourings – no salt but you can make a delicious broth using fresh herbs and spices, such as parsley, rosemary, sage, root ginger, chillies (the last two make it quite hot)
1.8 litres (3 pints) filtered water

Wash all the ingredients thoroughly, but don't peel. Leave any leaves attached. Chop roughly. Put the water into a large pan and add the vegetables – put them into the water as soon as you've chopped them so that they don't have time to be oxidized by exposure to the air. Bring up to the boil, cover and simmer for 45 minutes. Remove from the heat and allow to stand for a further 15 minutes. Strain the liquid into a clean pan and discard the vegetables.

Herb teas

These are a good way of increasing your fluid intake, especially if you feel cold and do not want to drink icy water. Herb teas have no tea in them – they're just pure herbs and in some cases spices too. You can either make your own with fresh herbs or buy them ready-made. Whether you use herbs or tea bags, you should let them infuse for at least 5 minutes in boiling water. There is an endless variety now available. Some of my favourites are:

Peppermint This is very soothing for the digestive system and also a good early-morning pick-me-up.

Chamomile Very calming and, when drunk last thing at night, should guarantee you a good night's sleep.

Ginger Chop up some pieces of root ginger and steep for about 10 minutes in hot water. This calms the digestive system, expels gas and is very warming.

Rosehip This is sweet-tasting and contains vitamin C.

Ayurvedic These teas, made according to Indian Ayurvedic medicine, are spicy and delicious. There are different types for sleep, energy and even detox.

Water

The other mainstay of your detox is to drink plenty of water. You need about 1.8 litres (3 pints) a day every day of the Plan – and beyond. This will help flush the toxins out of your system at the greatest speed. Drink filtered or bottled water.

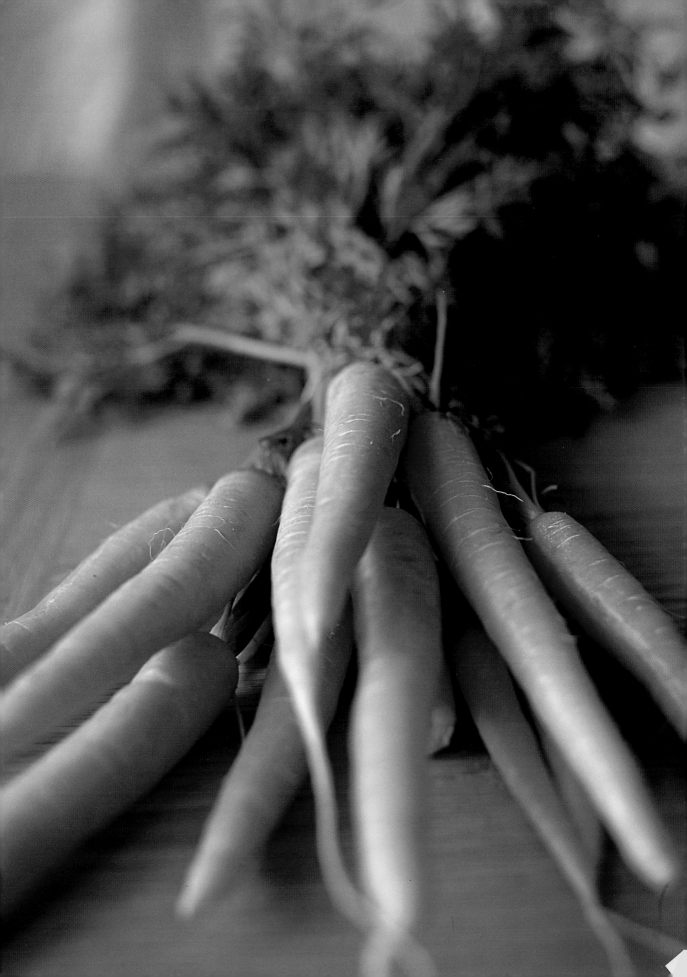

juice recipes

The important thing to remember when it comes to making juices is that they must be fresh – fresh ingredients and freshly made. Always drink the juice the moment you've made it. Don't be tempted to make double the quantity and store some for later; even sealed or in the refrigerator, it will start to lose vital nutrients.

These recipes are really just the beginning. Buy whatever looks freshest and best, and experiment. There's only one golden rule – with the exception of carrot and apple only, don't mix fruit and vegetables. (Carrot and apple will both mix with just about anything.) All the recipes make one large glassful.

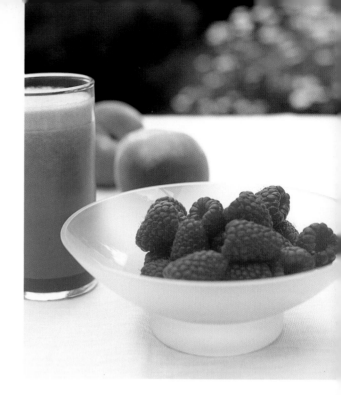

THE ULTIMATE DETOX JUICE
If I had to pick one juice as the best all-rounder for cleansing, immune boosting and simply being delicious, it would have to be this one.
4 carrots
2 green apples

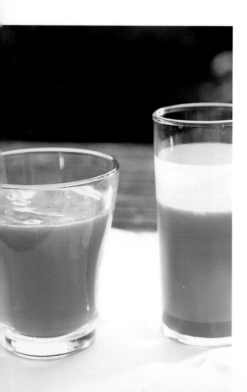

fruit juices

I've left out citrus fruits here as they have a very powerful scouring effect, and during a fast they are too harsh on the system.

APPLE JUICE
Apple juice is exceptionally high in minerals and vitamins and is a great cleanser. It combines with just about any other fruit brilliantly.
3 or 4 apples, depending on size

APPLE AND PEAR
Both are sweet and high in vitamins and minerals. Pear can be used as a mixer with other fruits if you have no apples.
2 apples
2 pears

APPLE AND WATERMELON
Watermelon is very cleansing, and if you juice the rind too you increase its nutritional value.
1/2 watermelon
2 apples

APPLE AND GRAPE
Grape juice has a lovely sweet taste and a thick consistency. It's also very cleansing.
small bunch of grapes
2 apples

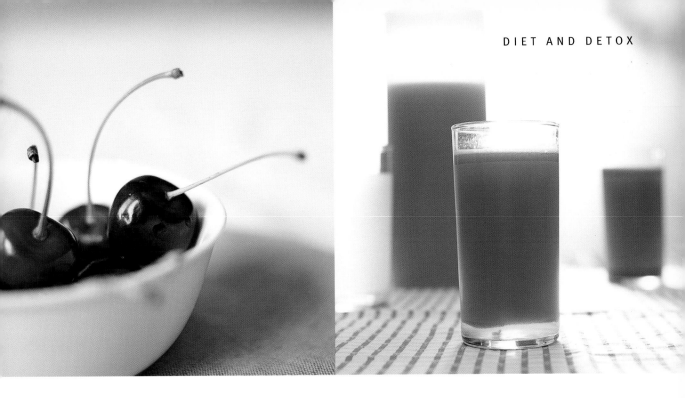

BERRIES AND APPLE

This one tastes as if summer has been poured into a glass!
small punnet of strawberries
small punnet of raspberries
2 apples

RHUBARB AND APPLE

The rhubarb stimulates the bowel, so it's good for constipation.
2 sticks rhubarb
3 apples

RASPBERRY AND PEACH

A thick, sweet, restorative juice, particularly good if you are overtired or anaemic. If you find it too thick, add an apple or two.
small punnet of raspberries
2 peaches

CHERRY AND GRAPE

A time-consuming juice to prepare, as you have to pick the grapes off the stalk and stone the cherries – but delicious when you've finished.
125 g (4 oz) cherries
small bunch of grapes

PINEAPPLE, MANGO AND PAPAYA

Wonderfully exotic and sweet, this is also an excellent energy booster, so it is good if you're feeling stressed or tired.
¹/₂ pineapple
1 mango
1 papaya

MELON JUICE

This is refreshing and delicious but not a good mixer, as it whizzes through the system. It is very easy to digest as a fruit to break the fast, too.
¹/₂–1 melon, depending on size

CRANBERRY, APPLE AND BANANA

Bananas actually yield very little juice but the flavour is so deliciously strong it overpowers the bitter cranberries. The latter are good for the kidneys.
125 g (4 oz) cranberries
2 bananas
2 apples

TOMATO JUICE

A delicious bright red juice, best drunk on its own.
6 tomatoes

vegetable juices

The vegetable juices are not so deliciously sweet as the fruit juices but they have a much more powerful cleansing and healing effect. The right combinations can be very palatable, too, but you need to consider the taste of the ingredients. Don't mix lots of very strong-tasting vegetables together – you won't be able to drink the result. I will always remember the day I tried juicing watercress. Because I love it so much in salads, I thought I'd try the juice neat. It brought tears to my eyes and nearly blew my head off. So if you are using vegetables that are very peppery or bitter, add carrots or cucumber as well to dilute and sweeten them.

CARROT, PARSLEY AND CUCUMBER

The ultimate diuretic! Parsley has a very strong taste, so you should use only a small amount.

handful of parsley
$1/_3$ cucumber
3 carrots

CARROT, BEETROOT AND CUCUMBER

Beetroot is one of the best juices for building up the number of red corpuscles in the blood. This is a very good juice if you suffer from anaemia or heavy periods. Use the tops of the beetroot, too.

2 carrots
1 beetroot (uncooked)
$1/_3$ cucumber

WATERCRESS, CARROT AND CELERY

Watercress is a powerful intestinal cleanser and adds spice – provided it is sufficiently diluted.

handful of watercress
3 carrots
2 celery sticks

DANDELION, CARROT AND TURNIP

Turnips are very peppery, so they need to be diluted with the milder carrots. Use the leaves, too.

handful of dandelion leaves
3 carrots
1 large or 2 small turnips

SPINACH, LETTUCE AND CARROT

Spinach is wonderfully cleansing, especially for the digestive system. This mix is one of the best suppliers of vitamins C and E and gives a great boost to the immune system and energy levels.

2 handfuls of spinach
$1/_2$ small lettuce
3 carrots

PARSNIP, POTATO AND CELERY

Potato juice is not particularly palatable on its own but it is an excellent detoxifier, while parsnip is believed to strengthen nails and celery is said to rejuvenate.

2 potatoes
2 parsnips
3 celery sticks

CELERIAC, ONION AND CUCUMBER

Celeriac has a delicious nutty flavour to balance the powerful taste of the onion, which on its own would certainly bring tears to the eyes. However, it has a powerful clearing effect on the sinus and the lungs, so it's excellent if you feel congested.

$1/_2$ celeriac
$1/_2$ small onion
$1/_2$ cucumber

FENNEL AND CUCUMBER

Fennel is very good for menstrual problems and for soothing nausea. It also clears the skin of blemishes – and tastes like Pernod!

1 head of Florence fennel
$1/_2$ cucumber

WHITE CABBAGE AND CAULIFLOWER

A refreshing, pale green juice, rich in folic acid and vitamin C.

$1/_2$ small white cabbage
$1/_2$ cauliflower

REMEDIAL JUICES

Some juices are beneficial for specific ailments. It will, of course, be quite a long time before any effect is felt, but they can help with a number of chronic conditions, infections, low immunity and low energy.

APPLE A great cleanser and good for digestive upsets, water retention, coughs and fatigue.

ARTICHOKE 1–2 tablespoons daily of this bitter juice is good for the liver, and for rheumatism and arthritis.

BEETROOT Restorative during convalescence, good for building up energy.

BLACKBERRY Good for anaemia and sore throats.

CABBAGE Small quantities only for problems of the stomach and liver and bronchial infections.

CARROT Immune booster *par excellence*! Good for building up red blood corpuscles and the liver.

CUCUMBER A natural diuretic, which also improves hair and nails.

MANGO, PAPAYA, PEACH Good for stress and fatigue.

PINEAPPLE An excellent energy booster.

RASPBERRY, STRAWBERRY High in iron, good for anaemia and general cleansing.

CELERY Good for arthritis.

PARSLEY Another good diuretic and high in vitamins and minerals.

WATERCRESS Very rich in minerals, an excellent blood purifier and detofixier.

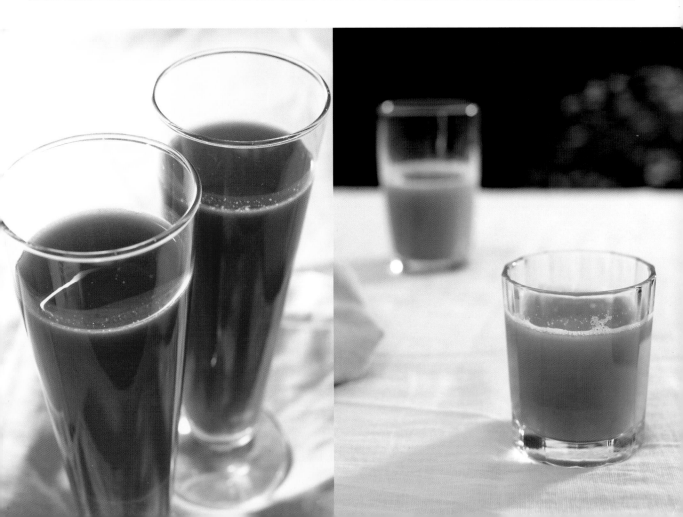

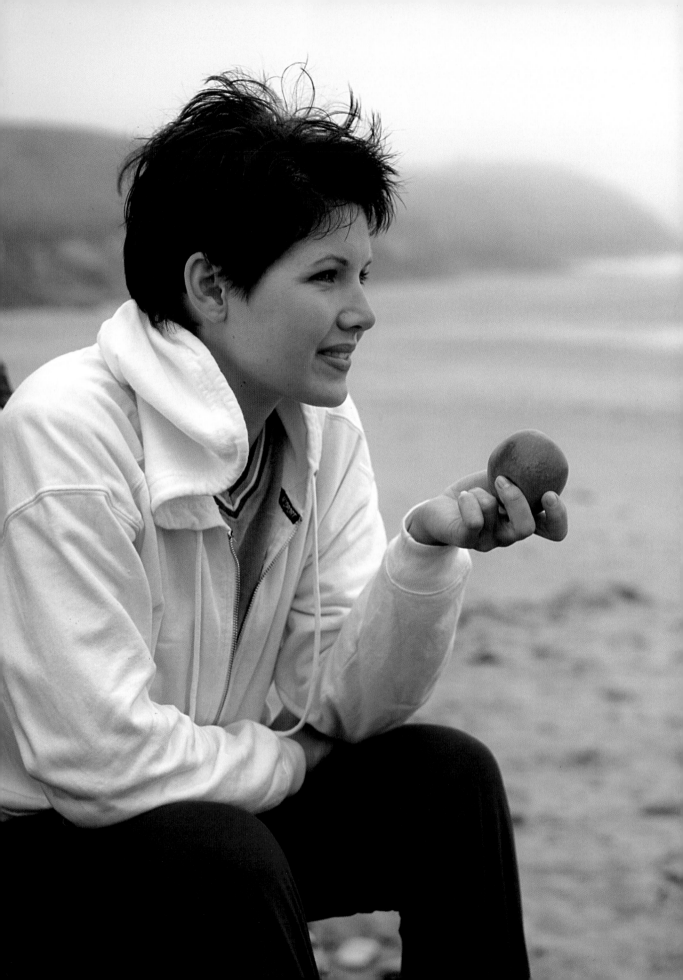

recipes

After the fast, the feast! Well, not exactly, but you will find that after your juice detox food is going to taste very good. The recipes here are super-healthy and will, in fact, continue the cleansing process you've started and set the standard for the kind of diet you can keep to in the future. Check in the week-by-week guides (see pages 110–15) for what to eat when.

You can eat as much as you want of the salad and soup meals. Remember to snack on as much fruit as you want during the day, as well as having at least two fresh juices daily, herb teas and, of course, lots of water.

breakfasts

Breakfast should give you the energy you need to start the day and keep on going all the way through. One of the best breakfasts is muesli – as invented by the famous Swiss physician and healer Max Bircher-Benner, and absolutely nothing like the kind you get from the supermarket shelf. It is not based on grains; the main ingredients are fruit and fruit juice.

Always have a fresh juice with your breakfast, even if you are eating fruit, and, as a hot drink, have herb tea. I find peppermint a good one to wake up to, but many people like fruit-based infusions or chamomile (a slice of lemon perks it up, too). Steer clear of the false buzz of the demon caffeine – this will be too much of a shock to your detoxing system.

All these breakfast recipes serve one.

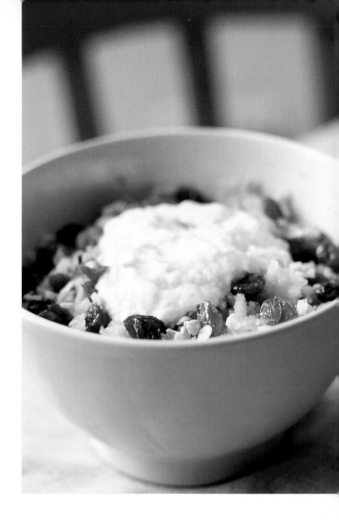

GINGERED APPLES

1 cooking apple
2 teaspoons honey
4 cloves
$\frac{1}{2}$ teaspoon ground ginger
live natural yogurt (optional)

Slice the apple and barely cover with water. Simmer for 10 minutes with the honey, cloves and ginger. Pour on some yogurt, if you like. For a change, substitute pear for the apple.

BIRCHER-BENNER MUESLI

2 tablespoons porridge oats
2 tablespoons raisins or sultanas
4 tablespoons apple or pineapple juice
1 apple or pear
1 tablespoon chopped mixed nuts
$\frac{1}{2}$ teaspoon ground ginger
1 teaspoon honey (optional)
2 tablespoons live natural yogurt

Soak the oats and raisins or sultanas overnight in the juice. Next morning, grate the apple or pear and mix into the oats together with the mixed nuts and ginger and, if you have a very sweet tooth, the honey. Pour the yogurt on top. This is a truly delicious breakfast and you can make any number of variations by adding different fruits in season.

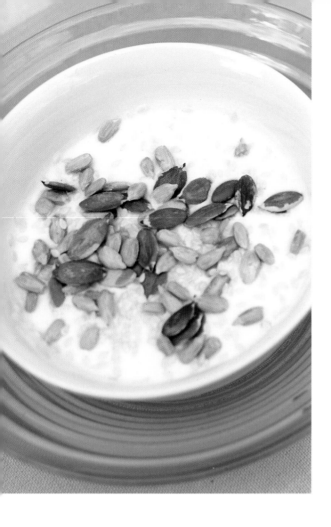

SEEDY YOGURT

25 g (1 oz) pumpkin, sesame and sunflower seeds
100 ml (3 ¹/₂ fl oz) live natural yogurt
1 teaspoon honey (optional)

Toast the seeds lightly or, alternatively, grind them up, then scatter them into the yogurt. If this isn't sweet enough for you, add a teaspoon of honey.

STUFFED FIGS

3 ripe figs
1 tablespoon ground almonds
25 g (1 oz) raspberries
1 teaspoon honey

Remove the stalks from the figs, make a criss-cross cut at the stalk end and carefully ease them open. Mix the almonds, raspberries and honey together and spoon into the open figs. You can serve this with a side dish of live natural yogurt.

YOGURT FRUIT

1 large (or 2 small) peach, pear or nectarine
25 g (1 oz) live natural yogurt
1 teaspoon toasted almonds, finely chopped
pinch of ground cinnamon
1 teaspoon honey (optional)

Slice the fruit into a bowl and pour on the yogurt. Sprinkle with nuts and cinnamon. If this isn't sweet enough, add a teaspoon of honey.

soups

Soup – the freshly made kind – is the perfect all-in-one food for health. These soups are packed with vitamins and minerals and they make substantial meals just on their own. Choose spicy soups if the day is chilly or if you're feeling under the weather (Immune Boosting Soup is good for this), substantial ones like Red Lentil or Sweet Potato if you're ravenous and fruit or herb soups when you want something refreshing.

All these recipes serve four people, as soups are something everyone enjoys. Any extra can be frozen for another day. I've added salt and pepper to all the recipes and the stock. However, salt should be kept to a minimum – try to reduce it a little each time you cook. Use as much pepper as you like, especially if you are experiencing headaches, congestion or cold-like symptoms.

PARSNIP AND CARROT SOUP

250 g (8 oz) parsnips, chopped
250 g (8 oz) carrots, chopped
1 onion, chopped
600 ml (1 pint) vegetable stock
salt and pepper
live natural yogurt, to garnish

Place the parsnips, carrots and onion in a large saucepan with the stock. Bring to the boil, season, cover and simmer for 15 minutes. Remove from the heat and allow to cool, then purée in a food processor until smooth, or rub through a sieve. Reheat the soup and serve garnished with yogurt.

VEGETABLE STOCK

3 potatoes
1 onion
2 leeks
2 celery sticks
2 carrots
1 head of Florence fennel
handful of herbs such as parsley, thyme, bay leaves
1.5 litres (2$\frac{1}{2}$ pints) water
salt and pepper

Simmer the vegetables and herbs with salt and pepper to taste in the water for about 1$\frac{1}{2}$ hours, skimming the surface regularly. Strain through a sieve and store in the refrigerator until required. If you are too short of time to make this stock, you can use bouillon powder or vegetable stock cubes instead.

YELLOW PEPPER SOUP

2 yellow peppers, cored and deseeded
2 tablespoons olive oil
1 small onion, finely chopped
600 ml (1 pint) vegetable stock
$\frac{1}{2}$ teaspoon curry powder
150 g (5 oz) potatoes
salt and pepper
1 teaspoon chopped fresh coriander, to garnish

Chop one of the peppers finely and the other roughly. Heat 1 tablespoon of the oil in a pan, add the onion and the roughly chopped pepper and cook for 5 minutes, stirring frequently. Pour the vegetable stock into the pan and add the curry powder and the potatoes. Bring to the boil and simmer for 40 minutes. In another pan, warm the remaining oil, gently cook the finely chopped pepper and set aside. Purée the mixture of onion, pepper and potatoes in a food processor until smooth, or rub through a sieve. Season to taste. Garnish with the finely chopped pepper and coriander.

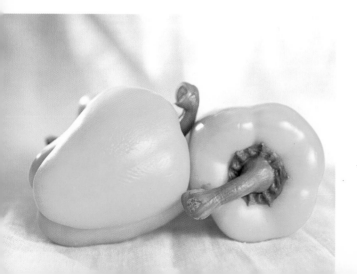

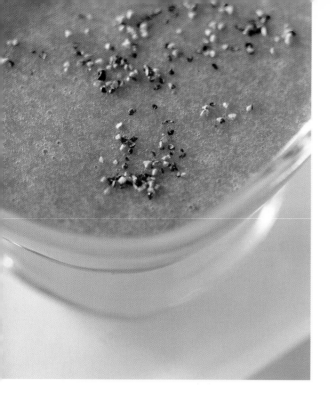

CHILLED FRESH FRUIT SOUP

2 apples, chopped
6 bananas, chopped
500 g (1 lb) strawberries, chopped
375 g (12 oz) pears, chopped
1 litre (1¾ pints) fresh orange juice
2 tablespoons lemon juice
300 ml (½ pint) fresh grapefruit juice
5–6 tablespoons clear honey
crushed peppercorns or mint and strawberries, to garnish

Place all the fruit in a food processor with 300 ml (½ pint) of the orange juice and blend. Add the lemon and grapefruit juice and honey and blend again. Pour the mixture into a large bowl, stir in the remaining orange juice, cover and chill in the refrigerator. Serve in a chilled bowl and garnish as preferred.

CHILLED TOMATO SOUP

2 tablespoons olive oil
1 small onion, chopped
1 garlic clove, chopped
750 g (1½ lb) tomatoes, skinned and finely chopped
600 ml (1 pint) vegetable stock
1 teaspoon chopped fresh oregano
¼ teaspoon celery salt
pinch of grated nutmeg
1 tablespoon Worcestershire sauce
150 ml (¼ pint) live natural yogurt
salt and pepper

To garnish
black olives
chopped fresh parsley

Heat the olive oil and gently cook the onion and garlic until transparent. Add the tomatoes to the pan and cook for a further 3 minutes. Pour in the stock and add the oregano, celery salt, nutmeg, Worcestershire sauce and salt and pepper. Bring to the boil then simmer, covered, for 40 minutes. Cool and blend in a food processor, or rub through a sieve. Stir in the yogurt and chill in the refrigerator for at least 3 hours. Garnish with olives and chopped parsley.

SWEET POTATO SOUP

2 tablespoons olive oil
2 carrots, chopped
1 onion, chopped
2 celery sticks, chopped
1 bay leaf
500 g (1 lb) sweet potatoes
250 g (8 oz) potatoes
600 ml (1 pint) vegetable stock
¼ teaspoon grated nutmeg
¼ teaspoon pepper
salt

Heat the oil in a saucepan and cook the carrots, onion and celery with the bay leaf over a low heat for 5–8 minutes, stirring frequently. Add the sweet potatoes, potatoes and stock and bring the mixture to the boil. Simmer, covered, for about 20 minutes. Remove the bay leaf. Blend the mixture in a food processor until smooth, or rub through a sieve. Return to the saucepan and add nutmeg, pepper and salt to taste.

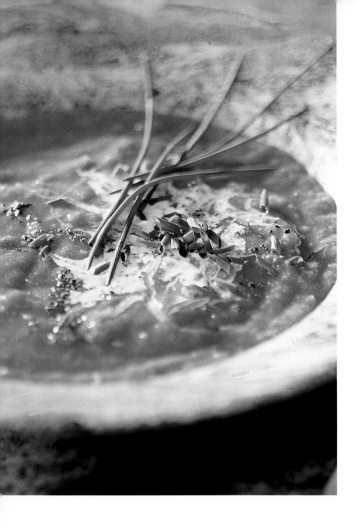

RED LENTIL SOUP

250 g (8 oz) split red lentils
1 leek, sliced
2 large carrots, sliced
1 celery stick, sliced
1 garlic clove, crushed
1 bay leaf
1.2 litres (2 pints) vegetable stock
$1/2$ teaspoon cayenne pepper
pepper

To garnish
live natural yogurt
finely chopped fresh parsley or chives

Put all of the ingredients except the garnish into a large saucepan, bring to the boil and simmer, covered, for 20 minutes. Allow the soup to cool, remove the bay leaf and purée the soup in a food processor until smooth, or rub through a sieve. Reheat, season with more pepper if necessary and serve in heated soup plates with the garnish.

IMMUNE-BOOSTING SOUP

500 g (1 lb) carrots, chopped
1 large potato, chopped
2 garlic cloves, chopped
1.2 litres (2 pints) vegetable stock
50 g (2 oz) chopped fresh parsley
1 teasoon chopped fresh sage
1 teaspoon chopped fresh thyme
1 teaspoon vegetable extract
$1/4$ teaspoon cayenne pepper

Place the carrots, potato and garlic in a large saucepan, add the stock and bring to the boil. Add all the herbs and spices, reduce the heat, cover and simmer for 20 minutes. Blend in a food processor until smooth, or rub through a sieve. Reheat and check the seasoning.

PARSLEY SOUP

150 g (5 oz) flat-leaf parsley, plus extra to garnish
600 ml (1 pint) water
2 tablespoons olive oil
1 onion, chopped
425 g (14 oz) potatoes, scrubbed and cut into 1 cm
    ($1/2$ inch) strips
$1/4$ teaspoon grated nutmeg
salt and pepper

Place the parsley in a saucepan, add the water and bring to the boil. Cover and simmer for 30 minutes. Rub the parsley through a sieve set over a large bowl. Discard any parsley left in the sieve. Heat the oil in a saucepan and cook the onion for 2–3 minutes, then add the parsley liquid and the potatoes. Bring to the boil, then lower the heat and simmer, covered, for 15–20 minutes. Add the nutmeg and salt and pepper to taste, and serve with a few parsley leaves as garnish.

CHICKPEA AND WATERCRESS SOUP

2 tablespoons olive oil
1 onion, chopped
500 g (1 lb) fresh spinach
1.2 litres (2 pints) vegetable stock
250 g (8 oz) potatoes, scrubbed and chopped
1 teaspoon lemon juice
pinch of grated nutmeg
150 ml (¼ pint) live natural yogurt
salt and white pepper

Heat the oil in a saucepan, add the onion and cook over a moderate heat until soft but not golden. Add the spinach to the pan and cook until it is soft. Pour in the stock, add the potatoes, lemon juice, nutmeg and salt and pepper and bring to the boil. Cook, partially covered, for 10–12 minutes. Blend in a food processor until smooth, or rub through a sieve. Reheat and add the yogurt, but do not let the soup boil.

COURGETTE SOUP WITH FRESH GINGER

2 tablespoons olive oil
250 g (8 oz) onions, chopped
1.5 kg (3 lb) small courgettes, thickly sliced
600 ml (1 pint) vegetable stock
1 tablespoon grated fresh root ginger
pinch of grated nutmeg
250 g (8 oz) potatoes, scrubbed and chopped
salt and pepper
live natural yogurt, to garnish

Heat the oil in a saucepan and cook the onions until soft but not golden. Add the courgettes and cook over a low heat for 5 minutes, stirring frequently. Add the stock, ginger and nutmeg, with salt and pepper to taste. Bring to the boil and add the potatoes. Simmer, partially covered, for 20 minutes. Blend in a food processor until smooth, or rub through a sieve. Reheat gently and serve garnished with a swirl of yogurt.

MUSHROOM AND MANGETOUT SOUP

50 g (2 oz) wholemeal flour
1 garlic clove, crushed
1 teaspoon chopped fresh thyme
1.2 litres (2 pints) vegetable stock
1 tablespoon olive oil
2 teaspoons vegetable extract
250 g (8 oz) mushrooms, sliced
250 g (8 oz) mangetout
50 g (2 oz) chopped fresh parsley

Make a paste of the flour with a little water. Add the garlic and the thyme. Heat the mixture over a low heat, slowly adding the stock and the oil and stirring continuously. Add the vegetable extract, mushrooms, mangetout and parsley and bring to the boil. Cover and simmer for 15 minutes, then blend in a food processor or rub through a sieve.

HEALTHY FISH SOUP

50 g (2 oz) wholemeal flour
2 teaspoons soy sauce
1 tablespoon olive oil
4 tablespoons lemon juice
1.2 litres (2 pints) vegetable stock
250 g (8 oz) turnips, chopped
250 g (8 oz) Florence fennel, chopped
1 onion, sliced
1 teaspoon cayenne pepper
350 g (12 oz) white fish, flaked

In a large saucepan, make a paste with the flour, soy sauce, olive oil, lemon juice and a little of the stock. Gradually add the rest of the stock over a low heat and bring the mixture slowly to the boil, stirring continuously. Add the turnips, fennel, onion and cayenne pepper to the soup and simmer for 10 minutes. Add the fish and cook for another 15 minutes.

salads

The key to a good salad is always to choose the freshest possible ingredients. Wash all leaves thoroughly in cold water and use a salad spinner so they're at their crispest for eating. All salads based on leaves can have added sprinkles. Lightly toast a mixture of sunflower, pumpkin and sesame seeds and scatter them over the top of your salad for a super-rich mix of essential oils and minerals. All the recipes here serve four so you can share your meal with friends or family. Reduce the quantities if you are making a salad for yourself – don't try to store some for later, it just won't be the same.

LEMON YOGURT DRESSING
Makes 175 ml (6 fl oz)

150 ml (¼ pint) live natural yogurt
1 tablespoon lemon juice
2 teaspoons chopped fresh mixed herbs
salt and pepper

Place all the ingredients in a bowl and whisk with a fork until well blended. Cover with clingfilm and chill in the refrigerator until ready to serve.

TARRAGON AND LEMON DRESSING
Makes about 75ml (3 fl oz)

2 tablespoons tarragon vinegar
1 teaspoon concentrated apple juice
1 teaspoon finely grated lemon rind
¼ teaspoon Dijon mustard
1 tablespoon chopped fresh tarragon
5 tablespoons olive oil
salt and pepper

Combine the vinegar, apple juice, lemon rind, mustard and tarragon in a small bowl. Add salt and pepper to taste. Stir to mix, then gradually whisk in the oil. Alternatively, put all the ingredients in a screw-top jar, close the lid tightly and shake well.

GUACAMOLE AND CRUDITES

1 avocado, stoned and mashed
1 tablespoon fresh lime or lemon juice
1 chilli, cored, deseeded and finely chopped
2 ripe tomatoes, finely chopped
2 tablespoons finely chopped onion
2 tablespoons chopped fresh coriander
1 garlic clove
pepper

Crudités
selection of raw vegetables, such as celery, red or green peppers, radishes, cauliflower, broccoli, carrots, fennel, chicory, cut into sticks or bite-size pieces

Mix the guacamole ingredients together in a bowl and serve with the crudités.

SWEET MUSTARD DRESSING
Makes 75 ml (3 fl oz)

3 tablespoons olive oil
2 tablespoons wholegrain mustard
1 tablespoon clear honey
1 teaspoon lemon juice
salt and pepper

Place all the ingredients in a small bowl and whisk with a balloon whisk or fork until thoroughly blended. Alternatively, put all the ingredients in a screw-top jar, close the lid tightly and shake until thoroughly combined.

MUSHROOM, COURGETTE AND TOMATO SALAD

6 large mushrooms, sliced
4 courgettes, sliced
4 tomatoes, sliced
1 teaspoon chopped fresh basil
1 bunch of watercress

Place the mushrooms, courgettes and tomatoes in a salad bowl and sprinkle with basil. Arrange sprigs of cress around the edge and serve with one of the dressings on this page.

RED LEAF SALAD

250 g (8 oz) medium soft goat's cheese (without rind) or
    cream cheese
40 g (1½ oz) pecan nuts, finely chopped
2 tablespoons paprika
175 g (6 oz) mixed red salad leaves, such as red chicory, lollo
    rosso, red oakleaf, radicchio
small handful of nasturtiums, pansies or other edible flowers
½ red onion, thinly sliced
Lemon Yogurt or Sweet Mustard Dressing (see opposite)

Mix the cheese and pecan nuts in a small bowl and shape into
balls. Spread out the paprika on a baking sheet and roll the
cheese balls in it until they are coated. Chill for at least 20
minutes. Arrange all the leaves and flowers, add the onion
and spoon over the dressing. Add the cheese balls and serve.

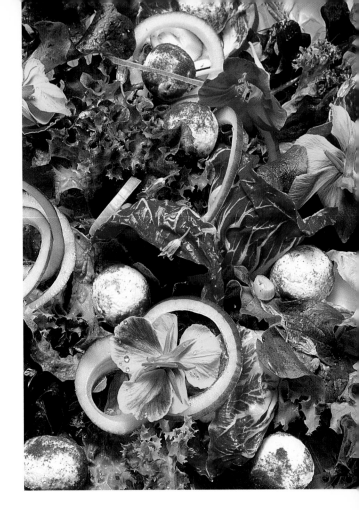

BULGAR WHEAT SALAD

250 g (8 oz) bulgar wheat
475 ml (16 fl oz) boiling water
250 g (8 oz) frozen broad beans
½ cucumber
1 small red onion, chopped
4 tomatoes, skinned and chopped
2 tablespoons finely chopped fresh mint
250 g (8 oz) feta cheese, crumbled or diced
salt and pepper
Sweet Mustard Dressing (see opposite)

Put the bulgar wheat in a large bowl and pour the boiling
water over it. Stir well and leave to stand for about 30
minutes, by which time all the water should be absorbed.
Transfer to a serving dish and allow to cool. Put the frozen
broad beans into a pan of boiling water and blanch for
1 minute. Drain and cool under cold running water. Remove
their outer skins to show the bright green insides and add to
the bulgar wheat. Peel the cucumber and cut in half
lengthways. Scoop out the seeds with a teaspoon and dice
the flesh. Add this to the salad with the onion, tomatoes and
mint. Season and toss. Sprinkle with the feta cheese and
serve with the dressing.

COTTAGE GARDEN SALAD WITH STRAWBERRIES

250 g (8 oz) mixed salad leaves (such as nasturtium,
    dandelion, rocket, red oakleaf, frisé, lamb's lettuce), torn
    into large pieces
handful of fresh herb sprigs, including some with flowers
    (such as fennel, dill, chives, mint)
250 g (8 oz) small strawberries, hulled
Lemon Yogurt Dressing or Tarragon and Lemon Dressing
    (see opposite)
salt and pepper

Put the leaves in a salad bowl and scatter the herbs over
them. Halve the strawberries (or leave whole if they are very
small) and add to the bowl. Season and then spoon the
dressing over the top.

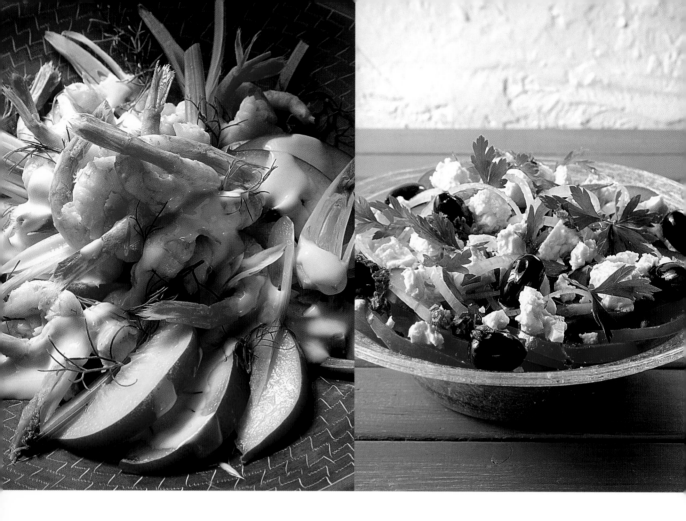

PRAWN AND FENNEL SALAD WITH PEACH

2 bunches of baby fennel, about 375 g (12 oz)
3 small ripe peaches, halved, stoned and sliced
1 bunch of watercress
375 g (12 oz) cooked peeled prawns
1 tablespoon lemon or lime juice
Lemon Yogurt Dressing (see page 52)
salt and pepper
pared rind of lemon or lime, to garnish

Remove all the frond-like tops from the fennel and roughly chop. Trim the fennel bulbs and slice them very thinly. Place in a shallow salad bowl with the chopped tops. Add the peaches and watercress. Toss the prawns in the lemon or lime juice and scatter over the salad. Season, then spoon the dressing over the salad and serve scattered with pared lemon or lime rind.

GREEK SALAD

4 small tomatoes, sliced
1 small onion, finely sliced
1 small cucumber, halved lengthways and cut into slices
1 green pepper, cored, deseeded and thinly sliced
125 g (4 oz) black olives
250 g (8 oz) feta cheese
flat-leaf parsley, roughly torn
juice of 1 lemon
pepper

Arrange the tomatoes overlapping slightly in concentric circles in a large serving bowl or on individual plates. Scatter the onion on top. Add the cucumber to the salad, along with the green pepper, black olives, feta cheese and parsley. Grind a little black pepper over the top, pour on the lemon juice and toss. With some wholemeal pitta bread, this can make a quite substantial main course.

MIXED LEAF SALAD WITH SPICED NUTS

175 g (6 oz) mixed salad leaves (such as lollo rosso, lamb's lettuce, rocket, young spinach)
small handful of chervil or dill sprigs
6 tablespoons Sweet Mustard or Lemon Yogurt Dressing (see page 52)

For the spiced nuts
2 tablespoons olive oil
50 g (2 oz) blanched almonds
50 g (2 oz) pecan nuts
2 tablespoons pine nuts
1 teaspoon chilli powder
1 teaspoon soy sauce
pinch of ground cumin
salt

Heat the oil in a pan, add all the other spiced nuts ingredients and cook for 1 minute. Tip into a baking tin and place under a preheated grill. Cook, turning frequently, for 5–10 minutes. Meanwhile, mix the salad leaves and herbs in a large salad bowl. Spoon the dressing over them, toss to coat the leaves and scatter the nuts over the top.

CONTINENTAL MIXED SALAD

1 red oakleaf lettuce, torn into bite-size pieces
1/2 head of frisé, torn into bite-size pieces
50 g (2 oz) rocket
50 g (2 oz) lamb's lettuce
small handful of fresh herb sprigs (such as chervil, dill, chives, basil, tarragon)
1 red onion, sliced
1 large avocado
1 tablespoon lemon juice
25 g (1 oz) toasted pine nuts
small handful of edible flowers (such as marigolds, nasturtiums, pansies)
Sweet Mustard Dressing (see page 52)
salt and pepper

Put the oakleaf lettuce and frisé in a large salad bowl with the rocket, lamb's lettuce, herbs and red onion. Peel, halve and stone the avocado. Roughly chop the flesh, place it in a small bowl with the lemon juice and toss gently to prevent discoloration. Add the avocado, pine nuts and edible flowers to the salad. Season and spoon the dressing over the salad.

FRENCH BEAN AND APRICOT SALAD

500 g (1 lb) French beans, topped and tailed
6 ripe apricots, halved, stoned and sliced
few sprigs of parsley
1 tablespoon chopped fresh tarragon
Sweet Mustard Dressing or Tarragon and Lemon Dressing (see page 52)
salt and pepper
handful of toasted sesame seeds, to garnish

Cook the beans in boiling water for 2–3 minutes. Drain in a colander, refresh under cold running water and drain again. Pat the beans dry with kitchen paper and place in a serving bowl. Add the apricots to the bowl with the herbs. Season, add the dressing and toss lightly. Garnish with toasted sesame seeds.

CELERIAC SALAD

250 g (8 oz) celeriac, grated or chopped into matchsticks
50 g (2 oz) toasted pine nuts
6 tablespoons of Lemon Yogurt Dressing (see page 52)
1 teaspoon horseradish sauce
salt and pepper

Mix the celeriac and nuts together. Combine the dressing and the horseradish sauce and mix in well, seasoning to taste.

main courses

These healthy, balanced main meals can be introduced in the final week of the 28-Day Vitality Plan – and, of course, they can form part of your long-term maintenance plan. You can have a main meal either at lunchtime or in the evening, depending on how it fits in best with your daily routine. For the final week, choose a soup or salad for the other meal. Again, all of these recipes serve four unless otherwise stated.

BABY CORN WITH ALFALFA

500 g (1 lb) baby corn cobs, halved lengthways
125 g (4 oz) alfalfa sprouts
5 tablespoons olive oil
1/2 onion, chopped
25 g (1 oz) flaked almonds
2 tablespoons white wine vinegar
1/2 teaspoon finely grated lemon rind
1 tablespoon chopped fresh parsley
salt and pepper

Drop the corn into a saucepan of boiling water and cook for 3–4 minutes. Drain and place in a large bowl with the alfalfa sprouts. Heat 2 tablespoons of oil in a small frying pan, add the onion and cook for about 3 minutes. Remove the onion from the pan. Add the almonds to the pan and cook, stirring, for 1–2 minutes until lightly browned. Return the onion to the pan with the remaining ingredients, including the remaining olive oil, stir well and add to the bowl of corn and alfalfa. Toss lightly.

STEAMED VEGETABLES WITH GINGER

250 g (8 oz) brown rice
3 carrots, sliced into thin rounds
4 tablespoons tomato purée
75 g (3 oz) cauliflower florets
75 g (3 oz) broccoli florets
2 small courgettes, sliced into thin rounds
3.5 cm (1 1/2 inch) piece of root ginger, cut into thin strips
4 tablespoons live natural yogurt, to garnish

Cook the rice according to the instructions on the packet. While the rice is cooking, put all of the ingredients except the yogurt in a steamer and steam for 7 minutes until tender. Drain the rice, arrange on plates and place the vegetables on top. Drizzle the yogurt over the vegetables.

VEGETABLE HOT-POT

4 carrots, sliced
4 parsnips, sliced
2 large courgettes, sliced
2 turnips, sliced
2 red or green peppers, cored, deseeded and coarsely chopped
2 onions, sliced
2 large tomatoes, skinned and coarsely chopped
600 ml (1 pint) Vegetable Stock (see page 48)
1 bay leaf
1 tablespoon chopped fresh parsley
1 teaspoon chopped fresh thyme
1 teaspoon chopped fresh marjoram
dash of soy sauce
salt and pepper

To garnish
4 tablespoons live natural yogurt
handful of toasted sesame, pumpkin and sunflower seeds

Place all the vegetables, the stock, the herbs and seasonings in a flame-proof casserole. Bring to the boil, skim, then cover and cook gently for about 25 minutes. Serve in individual bowls. Spoon the yogurt over and sprinkle with seeds.

STIR-FRIED VEGETABLES

1 tablespoon olive oil
125 g (4 oz) bamboo shoots, thinly sliced
50 g (2 oz) mangetout
125 g (4 oz) carrots, thinly sliced
50 g (2 oz) broccoli florets
handful of pine nuts
125 g (4 oz) fresh bean sprouts
1 teaspoon sweet soy sauce
1 tablespoon water

Heat the oil in a wok or frying pan and add the bamboo shoots, mangetout, carrots, broccoli florets and pine nuts, and stir-fry for about 1 minute. Add the bean sprouts and soy sauce and stir-fry for 1 further minute, adding water if necessary.

BAKED TROUT WITH DILL AND WATERCRESS
Serves 2

1 onion, chopped
2 garlic cloves, crushed
50 g (2 oz) watercress
2 x 200 g (7 oz) trout
1 tablespoon olive oil
4 sprigs of dill
salt and pepper

Place the onion and garlic in the top part of a steamer. Steam for about 5 minutes, season, add half the watercress and cook gently for 1 minute. Cut 2 double sheets of kitchen foil or greaseproof paper large enough to enclose the trout individually. Divide the onion mixture equally between the two. Clean the trout and brush with olive oil. Sprinkle inside and out with salt and pepper. Place one trout on top of the onion mixture on each piece of foil or paper and top with dill. Fold the foil or paper over the fish and wrap loosely, securing the sides and ends with a double fold. Place the parcels on a baking sheet and cook in a preheated oven, 180°C (350°F), Gas Mark 4, for 20 minutes. Remove the fish from the foil or paper and serve garnished with the remaining watercress.

HOT SCALLOP SALAD

8 large fresh scallops
3 tablespoons olive oil
$\frac{1}{2}$ small red pepper, cored, deseeded and cut into matchsticks
Sweet Mustard Dressing (see page 52)
1 tablespoon chopped fresh parsley
125 g (4 oz) rocket, roughly torn
$\frac{1}{2}$ small head frisé, roughly torn
2 spring onions, finely shredded
salt and pepper

Remove the corals from the scallops and set aside. Trim the white parts and cut each in half horizontally. Using a sharp knife, lightly score each scallop piece in a lattice pattern. Heat the oil in a large frying pan, add the scallops and the corals and cook, stirring, for 3–4 minutes, until opaque. Use a slotted spoon to transfer them to a plate. Add the red pepper to the pan and cook for 1 minute. Pour the dressing into the pan and heat, stirring in the parsley. Return the scallops to the pan and season. Put the salad leaves on individual plates and scatter the spring onions over the top. Finally, spoon on the warm scallop mixture.

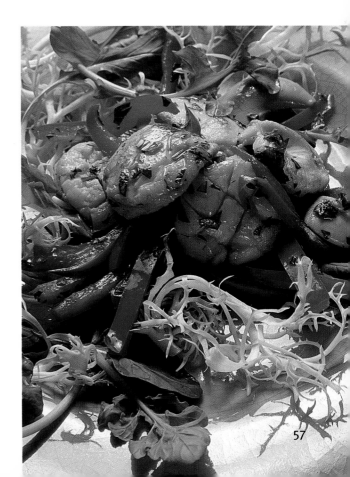

CHICKEN TANDOORI

4 skinned chicken breasts
1 garlic clove, crushed
1 tablespoon tandoori powder
300 ml ($\frac{1}{2}$ pint) live natural yogurt
onion slices, to garnish

Make incisions in the chicken flesh and rub with garlic. Place the chicken in a large, shallow bowl. Mix the tandoori powder with the yogurt and toss the chicken in the mixture. Place in the refrigerator to marinate for 3 hours. Heat the grill to moderate. Remove the chicken from the marinade and place on the grill rack. Grill for about 20 minutes, or until the chicken is cooked through, turning frequently and basting with the marinade. Transfer to a heated serving dish, garnish with onion slices and serve immediately.

PEPERONATA WITH WHOLEMEAL NOODLES

2 tablespoons olive oil
1 large onion, thinly sliced
1 large garlic clove, crushed
2 red peppers, cored, deseeded and cut into strips
2 green peppers, cored, deseeded and cut into strips
375 g (12 oz) tomatoes, chopped
1 tablespoon chopped fresh basil
175 g (6 oz) wholemeal noodles
salt and pepper
sprigs of fresh basil, to garnish

Heat 1 tablespoon of the olive oil in a deep frying pan. Add the onion and garlic to the pan and cook until the onion is soft but not coloured. Add the peppers, together with the tomatoes, the basil and seasoning. Cover and cook gently for 10 minutes. Remove the lid from the pan and cook over a fairly high heat until the moisture has mostly evaporated. Meanwhile, cook the noodles in plenty of boiling salted water until just tender. Drain and toss in the remaining olive oil. Season and divide among four plates, spooning the hot peperonata on top. Garnish with sprigs of fresh basil.

PASTA WITH TOMATO SAUCE

2 tablespoons olive oil
1 onion, chopped
1 garlic clove, crushed
375 g (12 oz) plum tomatoes, skinned and chopped
2 tablespoons tomato purée
a few black olives
handful of torn basil leaves
250 g (8 oz) wholemeal pasta
25 g (1 oz) grated Parmesan cheese (optional)
salt and pepper

Heat 1 tablespoon of the oil in a large frying pan. Sauté the onion and garlic gently over a low heat until tender. Add the tomatoes and the tomato purée. Cook over a gentle heat and allow the mixture to thicken. Stir in the olives and basil and season with a little salt and plenty of pepper. Meanwhile, boil the pasta in salted water until *al dente*, drain and stir in the remaining olive oil and some pepper. Arrange the pasta on plates with the sauce on top and sprinkle with a little Parmesan, if liked.

PASTA WITH THREE HERB SAUCE

3 tablespoons chopped fresh parsley
1 tablespoon chopped fresh tarragon
2 tablespoons chopped fresh basil
1 tablespoon olive oil
1 large garlic clove, crushed
6 tablespoons vegetable stock
375 g (12 oz) wholemeal pasta
salt and pepper

Put the herbs, oil, garlic, stock and seasoning into a food processor and work until smooth. Cook the pasta in a large pan of salted boiling water for 10–12 minutes until just tender. Drain and heap into a warmed serving bowl. Pour the herb sauce over the pasta.

SMOKED TROUT AND PASTA

175 g (6 oz) pasta shells or bows
1 tablespoon olive oil
40 g (1 1/2 oz) flaked almonds
250 g (8 oz) broccoli, broken into florets
125 g (4 oz) frozen peas
250 g (8 oz) smoked trout fillets, flaked
125 g (4 oz) cherry tomatoes, halved
salt and pepper
sprigs of dill or parsley, to garnish

Cook the pasta in salted boiling water until *al dente*, then drain in a colander. While the pasta is cooking, heat the oil in a small pan and cook the almonds for 1 minute until browned. Tip into a large bowl. Add the cooked pasta to the bowl and mix with the almonds. Add the broccoli and peas to a large pan of boiling water and cook for just 3 minutes so that the broccoli is still crunchy. Add to the bowl of pasta. Finally, add the trout and the cherry tomatoes. Season with a little salt and pepper and garnish with dill or parsley.

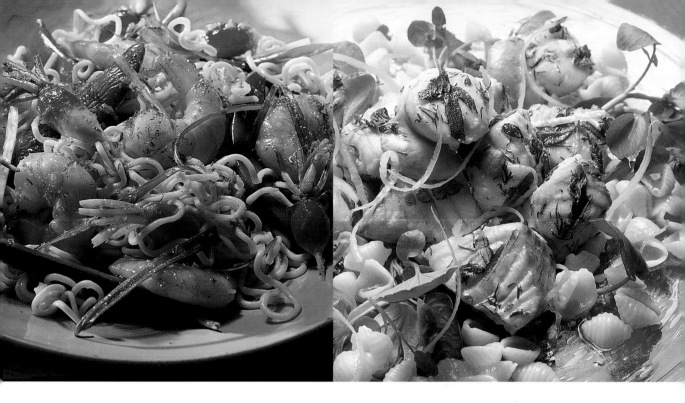

CHINESE NOODLES AND PRAWNS

175 g (6 oz) Chinese noodles
6 spring onions, cut into short lengths and finely shredded
small bunch of radishes, sliced or left whole
175 g (6 oz) sugar snap peas, topped and tailed
175 g (6 oz) cooked peeled prawns
salt and pepper

For the sauce
2 teaspoons grated fresh root ginger
1 garlic clove, crushed
finely grated rind and juice of 2 limes
1 tablespoon clear honey
75 ml (3 fl oz) groundnut or grapeseed oil
2 tablespoons chopped fresh coriander
salt and pepper

First make the sauce. Combine the ginger and garlic in a bowl, then add the lime rind and honey. Season lightly. Add the lime juice to the bowl and beat well with a balloon whisk or wooden spoon. Pour in the oil and whisk. Put the bowl in a pan of boiled water and leave to heat through slightly.

Bring a saucepan of water to the boil, add the noodles, cover the pan and remove from the heat. Leave to stand for 5 minutes, then drain and transfer to a bowl. Add the spring onions and the radishes to the bowl of noodles. Bring a saucepan of water to the boil, add the sugar snap peas and blanch for 1 minute. Drain and add to the bowl, along with the prawns. Add the chopped coriander to the sauce, pour over the pasta mixture and mix lightly.

GRILLED SALMON AND SCALLOPS

500 g (1 lb) salmon steak
500 g (1 lb) shelled large scallops
175 g (6 oz) pasta shells
175 g (6 oz) mixed salad leaves such as frisé, red oakleaf, cos,
    lamb's lettuce, watercress, torn into bite-size pieces

For the marinade
125 ml (4 fl oz) light olive oil
pared rind of $^1/_2$ lemon
2 teaspoons chopped fresh oregano
1 tablespoon chopped fresh dill
salt and pepper

Mix all the marinade ingredients together and pour into a shallow dish large enough to hold the fish. Cut the salmon into chunks the size of the scallops. Thread the salmon and scallops alternately on to 4 long skewers. Arrange in the marinade, turning them to coat. Leave for 1$^1/_2$–2 hours, turning occasionally. Preheat the grill to hot. Remove the brochettes from the marinade and arrange in one layer on the grill rack. Grill for 8–10 minutes, turning frequently and basting with the marinade throughout. Meanwhile, cook the pasta in salted boiling water until *al dente*. Drain and put in a large serving bowl with the salad leaves. Remove the seafood from the skewers and pile on top of the pasta. Mix lightly and serve.

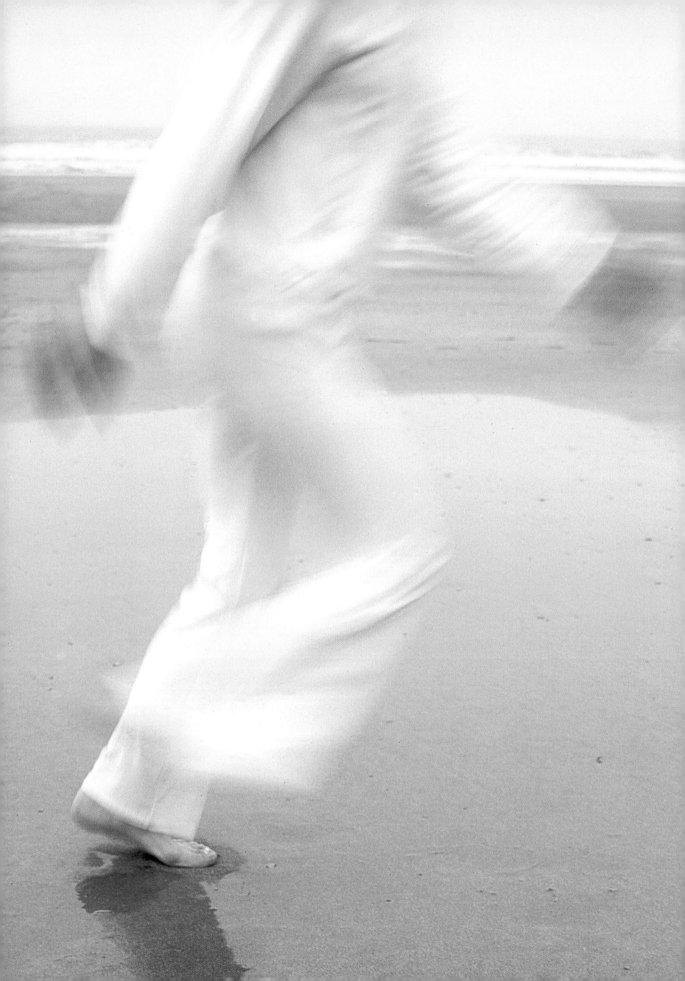

exercise

There isn't a wrong reason for wanting to get in shape – but there is a wrong approach. If you see your body as something you can starve, pummel and bully into shape, you will discover that unless you are ruthlessly determined you can find neither the time nor the discipline to maintain your regime. The next thing you know your old bad habits will have reasserted themselves and you will have lost the gains you made.

Exercise need not be a chore. The exercises given here are gentle and aim to stretch and tone your whole body – not to build up bulky muscles. As you progress through the 28-Day Vitality Plan, you will be conditioning your body and at the same time discovering you have more vitality. This is due to a hormone called noradrenalin (or norepinephrine) which is released each time you exercise. It is nicknamed the 'kick' hormone because this is precisely what it does – it gives you a natural high that makes you more alert and increases your sense of well-being, besides decreasing feelings of hunger. At the same time, exercise also raises the beta-endorphin levels in the body and these help you to relax and to sleep better. There's no doubt about it – our bodies deserve the benefits of exercise.

warm-up exercises

Before you start working on any specific area of the body to tone, shape or strengthen it, it is vital to warm up first. This prevents possible strains and injury, which are much more likely when your muscles are cold. These first exercises also loosen the shoulders, hips, ribs and the all-important spinal column.

ROLL DOWN

Start with the roll down on page 14 and perform the whole exercise 3 times.

SHOULDER CIRCLES

1 Stand with a good posture, your shoulders dropped and relaxed. Start to rotate the shoulders forwards. If you're doing it correctly, your arms will have turned so that your palms are facing towards you.

2 Continue the circle so that the shoulders lift up towards the ears then pull them down and back, so that your shoulder blades squeeze together. Make sure that at this point you don't arch the small of the back.

3 Finally, drop your shoulders right down. If you feel any tension in your neck, drop your head forwards onto your chest to relax the muscles. Do 3 circles and then another 3 in reverse.

PUSH ME-PULL YOUS

Stand with good posture, your feet about 45 cm (18 inches) apart. Clasp your fingers together in line with your chest, then pull them away from each other without actually letting go. You should feel the muscles of the upper arms working together with the pectorals as the chest opens. Repeat 8 times and then reverse the process, pushing the hands together 8 times. Your head should be lifted throughout and your neck long. If you feel any tension in the area, drop your head forwards onto your chest to relax the muscles.

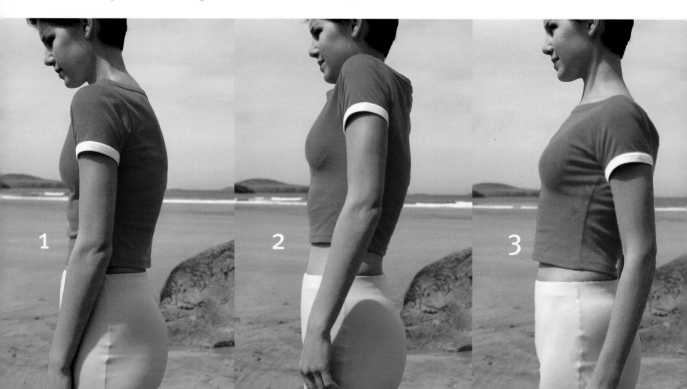

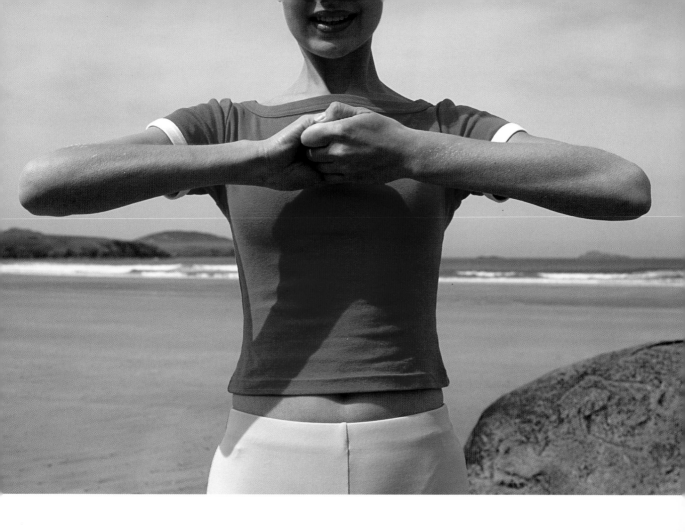

ARM STRETCHES

1 Standing with your feet about 45 cm (18 inches) apart, stretch alternate arms from the elbow upwards. Bend the knee on the same side as the arm you are stretching, shifting your body weight from side to side. The source of the arm stretch should be from the shoulder blade, with the shoulder well dropped down. This is not just an arm stretch – the top half of the body should be stretching up out of the waist. Repeat 16 times.

2 Now take alternate arms straight out to the side and repeat this movement 16 times.

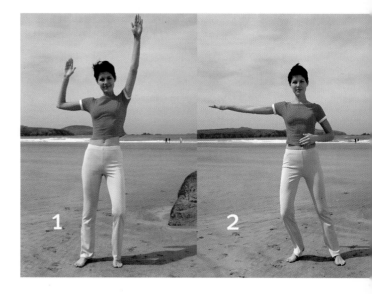

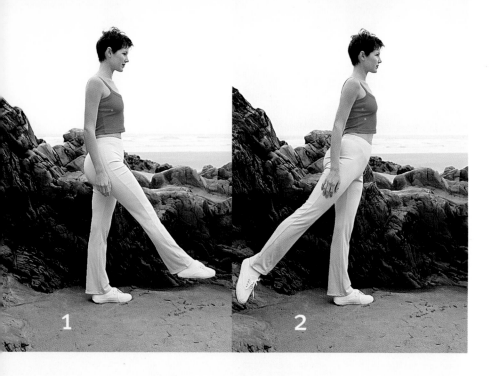

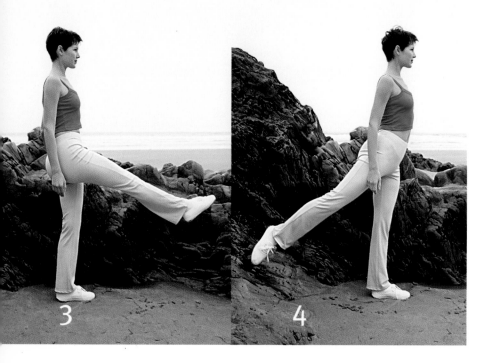

PLIES

1 & 2 Stand tall with your feet together, then bend your knees as much as you can without taking your heels off the floor. As you do this, feel your stomach muscles pushing back towards your spine and your spine growing longer – take care not to arch it. Do this 8 times.

3 & 4 Next, turn your feet out in a V shape. Make sure to keep your knees over your feet at all times – don't allow them to roll in as this could damage them. Bend your knees, feeling your thigh muscles turn out and your buttock muscles pull under. Bend 3 times, keeping your heels on the floor.

5 On the fourth bend, allow your heels to rise and go down as far as you can, keeping your back straight – you may want to hold on to a support to do this. Repeat the sequence twice more.

6 & 7 Finally, with your feet about 45 cm (18 inches) apart, turn your legs out from the hip sockets so your knees are over your feet. Bend in the same way as the previous pliés, keeping your heels firmly on the ground, with your thigh muscles turning out. Do not lift your heels at all. Do 4 slow pliés.

LEG SWINGS

1, 2, 3 & 4 These exercises warm up the hip socket. Stand with a good posture, one hand resting on a suitable support, such as chair back. Take the outside leg straight back and then forwards in a gentle swing. Repeat 16 times, raising the leg a little higher each time. Change sides and repeat with the other leg.

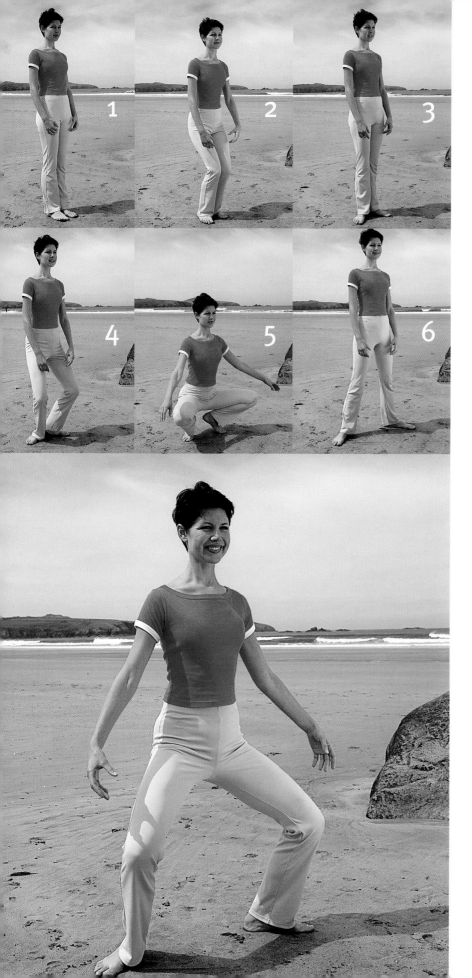

ROLL DOWNS

Finally, do three roll downs (see page 14). Your back should feel much looser now.

trim torsos

The stomach muscles are often some of the weakest in a woman's body, and we tend to make up for this fact by letting the back take the strain. Our backs can end up hunched, tense and overarched as a result – doing us a double disservice, as this results not only in bad posture but can lead to permanent injury, too. When you strengthen the stomach muscles, you take pressure off the back and get a flat tummy in the process.

If your stomach muscles start to bulge or quiver at any time during these exercises, you are attempting something that is as yet beyond them – so stop! When you are lying on your back, the lower your legs are towards the floor the more strain you will be putting on the stomach; lift them higher and the exercise will instantly become easier. When you are doing these exercises – and indeed all the time – try to think of the stomach muscles providing a natural girdle, keeping the body in a lifted, well-held posture.

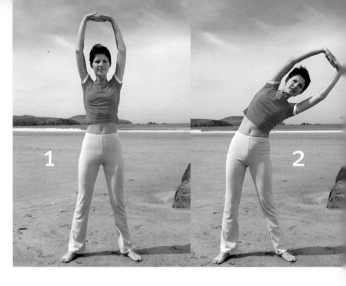

SIDE STRETCHES

1 With your feet hip-width apart and slightly turned out, lift your arms above your head and clasp your hands together, keeping your shoulders dropped.

2 In one smooth movement, looking straight ahead, drop down to the left, bending from the waist. Try to get low enough for your arms to be parallel with the floor. Come back to the centre and repeat on the right. Do 4–8 drops each side.

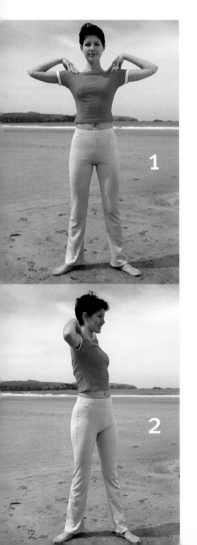

TORSO TWISTS

With these twists, it is important to remember that it is only the waist and upper body that turn – the hips stay absolutely still and facing the front.

1 Stand with your feet hip-width apart, feet slightly turned out and knees bent. Rest your hands lightly on your shoulders, elbows pointing straight out. Feel your back straight and your tailbone dropping down towards the floor.

2 Turn from the waist to look over your left shoulder. Do 16 turns and then repeat to the right.

UPPER BODY CIRCLES

This is a more complex version of the Torso Twists exercise.

1 Stand with your feet hip-width apart and slightly turned out, your arms raised, shoulders down and hands clasped.

2 Drop down to the left until your arms are parallel to the

floor, feeling the stretch all the way up your right side.

3 Now turn so that you are looking down at the floor, but keep your body on the same level. This calls for a lot of work from the stomach muscles.

4 Turn back so you are facing forwards again and then straighten up. Build up to 4 times each side.

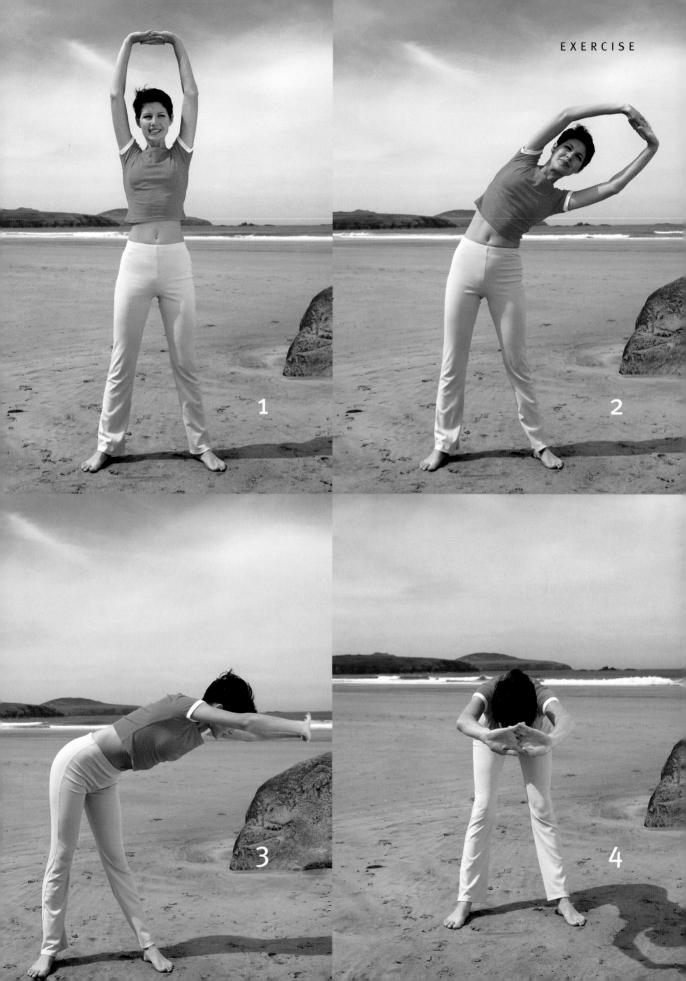

ROLL-UPS

This is a series of exercises that build up in difficulty, so start with the first one and only go on to the later ones as your muscles strengthen.

1 Lie on the floor with your legs stretched out and your arms at your sides, palms upwards. Pull your stomach muscles back into the floor, tightening your buttock muscles under you at the same time. This will cause your knees to bend slightly and your pelvis to tilt. Repeat 4 times.

2 In the second stage, repeat the pelvic tilt, this time moving your upper body off the floor, arms outstretched and parallel to the floor. Your head should come up last. Do not raise yourself far enough to make your stomach bulge or your shoulders tense. Repeat 4 times.

3 In the third stage, you begin as before and continue to raise your upper body until you are sitting straight up, arms stretched out in front, head and neck in a long line with your spine.

4 Now drop your head forward onto your chest and roll back down through the spine, holding on tight to the stomach muscles. Try to feel your back go down, vertebra by vertebra, lengthening out on the floor. Repeat 4 times.

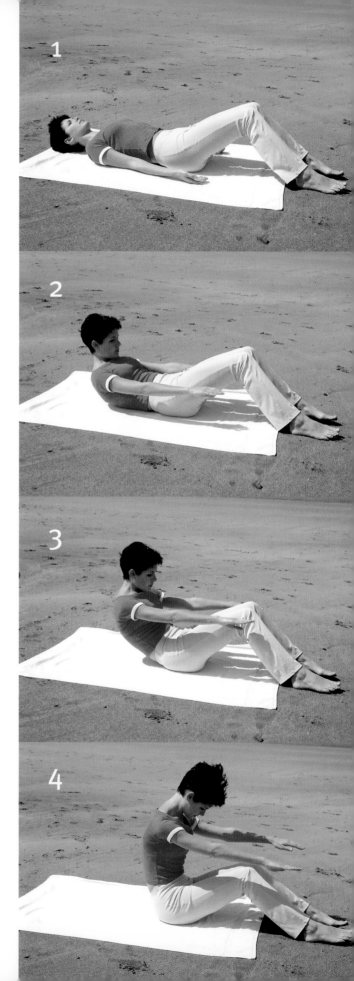

ROPE CLIMBING

This is quite a tough exercise for the abdominal muscles, so don't try it until you can do the first four exercises comfortably.

Start by lying on your back on the floor. Contract your stomach muscles so that you start to roll up until you are about halfway to a sitting position, knees bent, arms outstretched in front of you. Loosely clench your fists, then raise one arm above your head. Lower this arm again and, as you do so, raise the other one. This movement looks as if you are pulling on a rope. If the stomach muscles start to bulge out or quiver, stop. Repeat for 8 pulls.

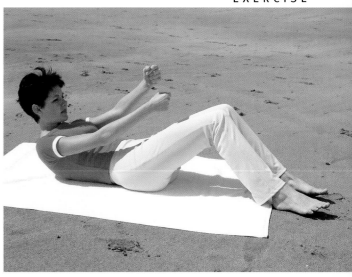

CROSSED FISTS

This is a continuation of the previous exercise – and another very tough one!

Start by lying on your back on the floor. Contract your stomach muscles so that you start to roll up until you are about halfway to a sitting position, knees bent, arms outstretched in front of you. With your hands in loose fists, cross and recross one above the other, raising your arms at the same time until they are reaching straight upwards. Make sure you don't tense your neck or shoulders as you do this. When you reach the top, reverse and come down in four crosses. Repeat the whole sequence 4 times up and down.

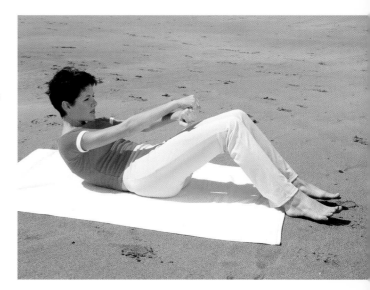

SCISSORS

Another tough one for the abdominals! If you're not ready for this, the small of your back will come off the floor – in which case, stop. Remember, the lower the legs, the harder the exercise.

Lie flat on the floor, arms by your side, then bend your knees into your chest and stretch your legs upwards. With your fingers resting just behind your ears, lift your head and shoulders off the ground and look up at your legs. Pull your stomach well in and if the exertion is too great raise your legs higher. Now scissor your legs, crossing them at the ankles, 16 times.

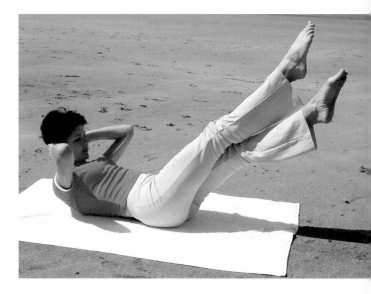

beautiful bottoms

The obsession that most women have about their bottoms is well documented. In fact, one of the problems with bottoms is that their muscles don't get much used in everyday life. Improving your posture will be a good start at waking those muscles up, while the following exercises will strengthen them, thus lifting and firming the buttocks.

BACK LEG LIFTS

1 Lie on your front, resting on your elbows. Bend your right leg slightly and keep the foot flexed. Raise the left leg and stretch it to its full extent, pointing the foot. You should be able to feel the leg muscles working right into the buttocks.

2 Do 16 lifts each side then repeat another 16 times with the foot flexed.

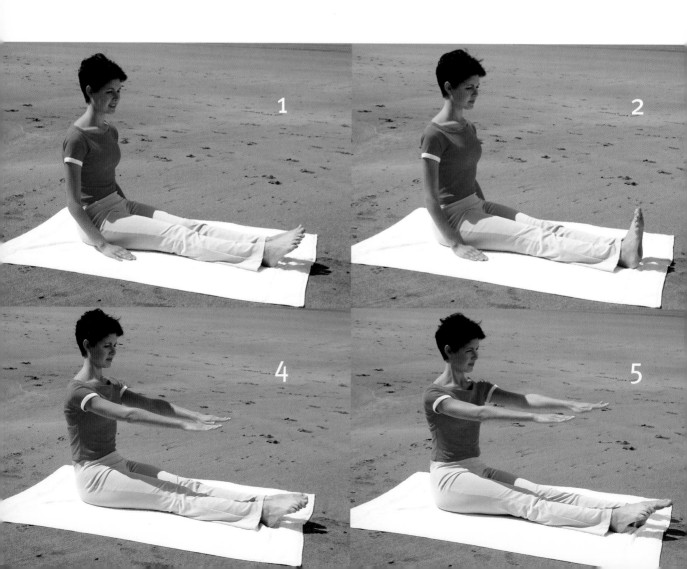

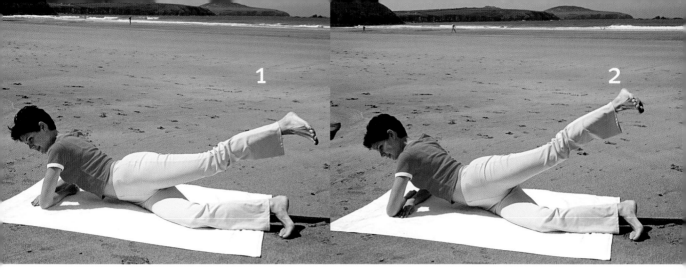

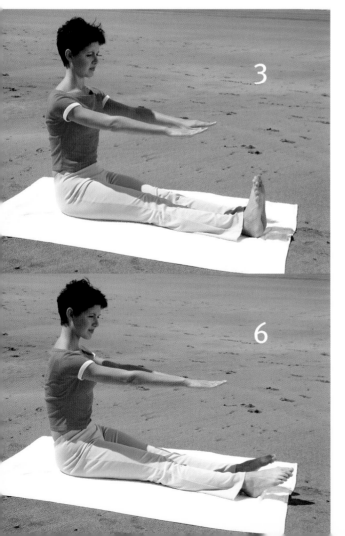

BUTTOCK AWARENESS

1 Sit on the floor, your legs stretched out in front, feet pointed. Your back should be perfectly straight, your arms beside you and hands on the ground.

2 Pull your buttock muscles tight beneath you – you should find you are sitting about 5 cm (2 inches) higher! Do this clenching and releasing 16 times.

3 & 4 Now, with your buttocks clenched and your arms straight out in front of you, point and flex your feet 16 times.

5 Finally, point your feet again and, sitting tall, move the left leg from the hip as if you are walking on your buttocks.

6 Alternate your legs so you walk 8 'steps' forwards and 8 back.

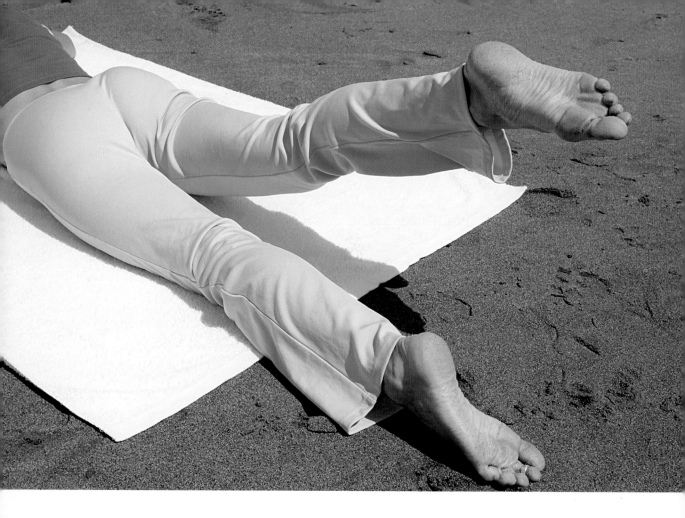

LEG CIRCLES

Lie flat on your front, your face on your arms. Raise one leg straight behind you and make 16 little circles with your pointed foot, clockwise and then anti-clockwise. Repeat with the other leg.

LEG STRETCHES

1 Lie face down on the floor, arms and legs stretched, feet about hip-width apart. Pull up your stomach muscles so that there is enough space to slide your hand between your stomach and the floor. Try to keep that pulled-up feeling throughout this exercise. Stretch out your left arm and right leg simultaneously, feeling the stretch right through your body – the stretch should lift your arm and leg about 15 cm (6 inches) from the ground. Repeat with the opposite arm and leg. Do the exercise 8 times on each side.

2 Now repeat 8 times with both arms and legs stretching at once.

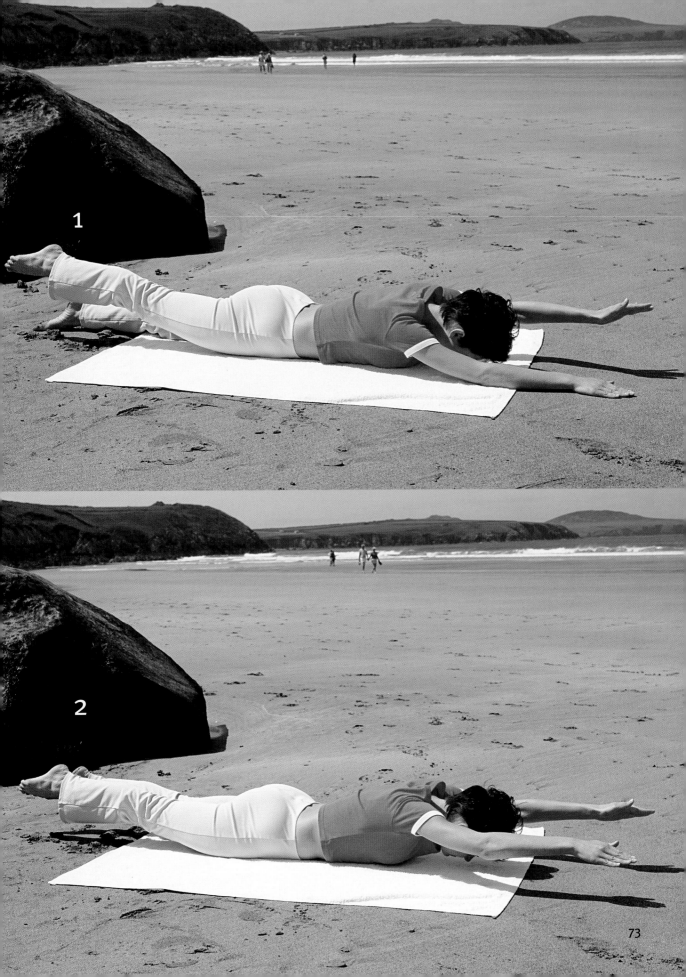

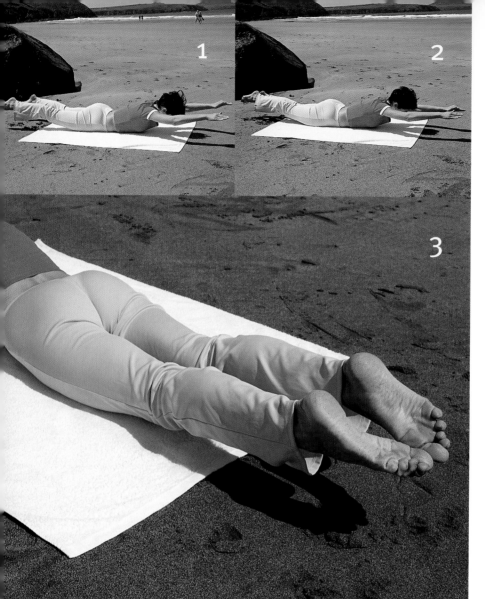

TURN-OUT

Stand up very tall, your upper body relaxed and your back absolutely straight. Turn out your legs from the hip sockets very slowly so that your feet form a 'V' shape. Don't take your feet too far – your knees should be over your feet at all times, not rolling inwards. At the same slow pace, draw your feet back to a parallel position. This exercise works the muscles of the buttocks and the inner and outer thighs. Repeat for 16 complete movements.

FOOT TAPPING

1, 2 & 3 Lie face down on the floor and stretch out your arms and legs, with your head and chest off the floor as well. Now tap the feet together, working up to 50 taps.

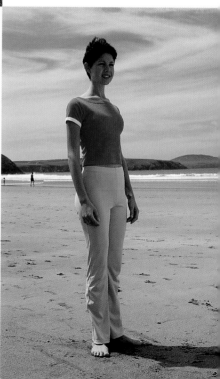

DEEP PLIES

The more slowly you do this exercise, the more effective it is. You may need to hold a support such as a chair back to one side to help you balance.

1 Stand tall with your feet about 45 cm (18 inches) apart, your legs turned out from the hips without trying to over-extend the turn-out in the feet or ankles.

2 Keeping your back straight, drop your tailbone down towards the floor, bending your knees but without taking your heels off the floor.

3 Squeeze your thighs together to straighten, pulling up the muscles in your buttocks and the backs of your thighs.

4 Keep on squeezing so hard that you rise up on to your toes. Come down in one slow, smooth movement and bend the knees into another deep plié. Repeat the whole sequence 4 times in all, changing sides if you are keeping your balance by holding a chair back.

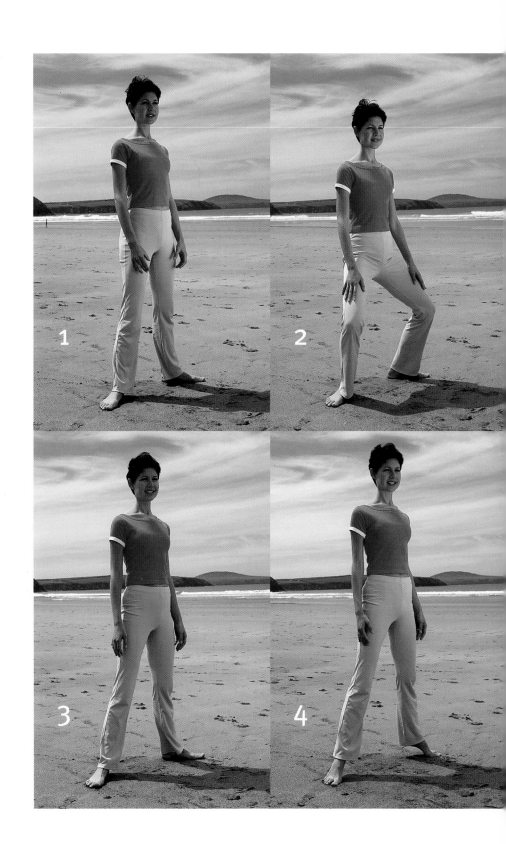

thigh trimmers

Let's face it – nobody wants to be pear-shaped. That bulge over the hips and the jodhpur thighs are not exactly appealing. Unfortunately, for most women, this is exactly where fat is most likely to accumulate, often with the 'orange-peel' effect of cellulite. This needs to be attacked on two fronts, the first being diet and the second being exercises that lengthen and strengthen. The exercises that follow do not build up bulky muscle – they are designed to elongate the legs. Where the leg is to stretch in an exercise, you should feel it pulled out to its full extent all the way from the hip socket to the pointed toes.

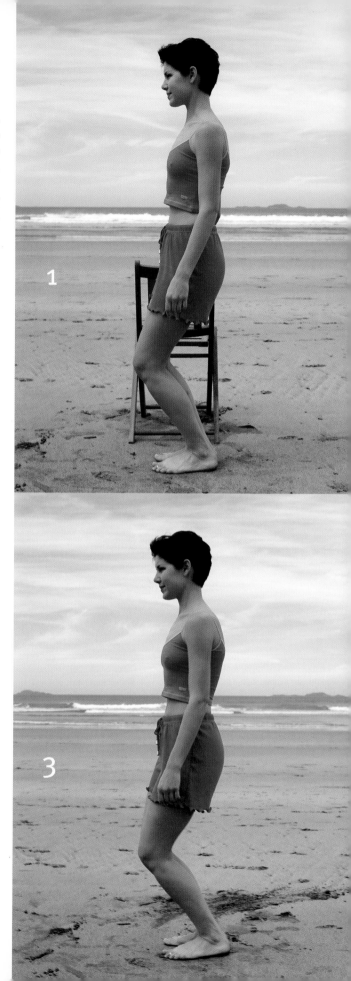

PARALLEL PLIES

These pliés strengthen the muscles at the front of the thighs, which not only gives your leg a firm, curved front but also protects the knees.

1 & 2 Stand tall with one hand resting on a chair back, feet together and facing forwards. Keeping your spine straight, bend your knees, dropping your tailbone directly down to the floor and moving in one piece, only peeling your heels off

the floor when you have to. Come back to standing and carry on upwards into a rise. Repeat for 4 pliés and rises on each side.

3 & 4 Move away from the chair but stand in the same lifted position. This time, as you bend, let your bottom stick out and aim to get your upper thighs parallel to the floor without lifting your heels. Swing your arms forward as you go down to help you balance. Repeat 16 times.

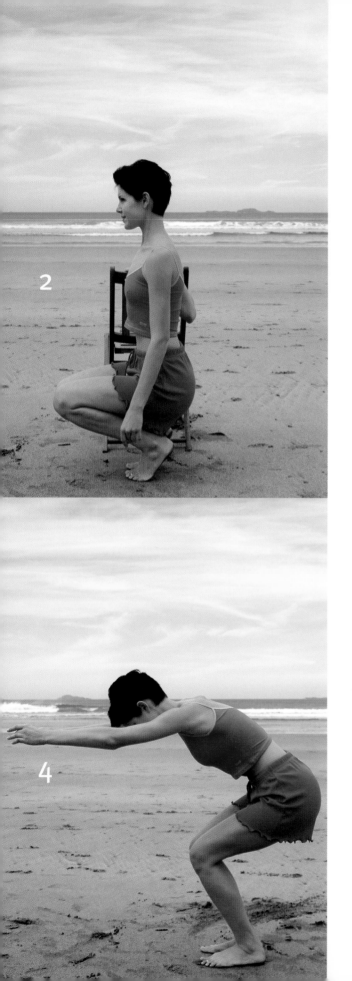

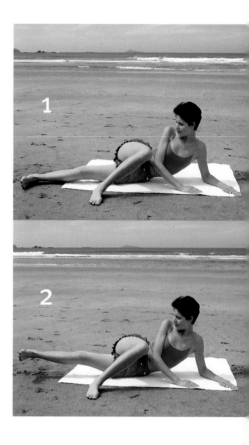

INNER THIGH LIFTS

1 Lie on your side, propped up on one elbow or lying down flat along an outstretched arm. Bring the top leg over you, bending your knee, and place the foot on the floor. Extend the lower leg and flex the foot.

2 Lift the lower leg about 15 cm (6 inches) off the floor 16 times. Now repeat for another 16 with your foot pointed. Repeat the whole exercise on the other side.

77

LEG LIFTS

1 Lie on your side, propped up on one elbow or lying down flat along an outstretched arm, as you prefer. Bend the lower leg and flex the foot so the heel is raised slightly off the ground. Flex the upper foot and push the heel away hard so the leg feels as if it is pulling out of the hip socket all the way through the exercise. Keep your back straight and your stomach held in.

2 Raise the leg and, from the raised position, do 16 small lifts.

3 Lower the leg and take it forwards so that it is at a right angle to your body.

4 Keeping the foot flexed, raise it 16 times. Finally, in the same position, make 16 small circles clockwise then 16 anti-clockwise. Repeat the whole exercise on the other side.

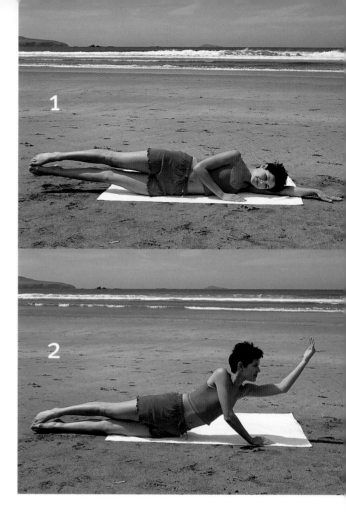

DOUBLE LEG LIFTS

This exercise works the legs and the stomach very hard!

1 Lie flat on your side with your lower arm extended above your head. Point your

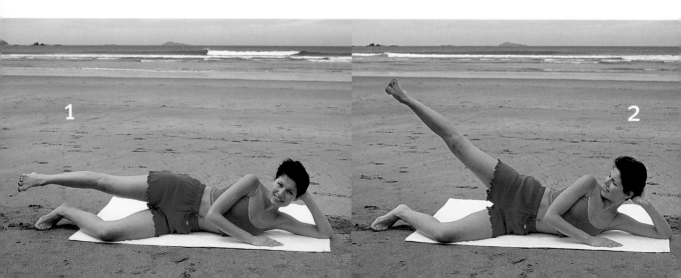

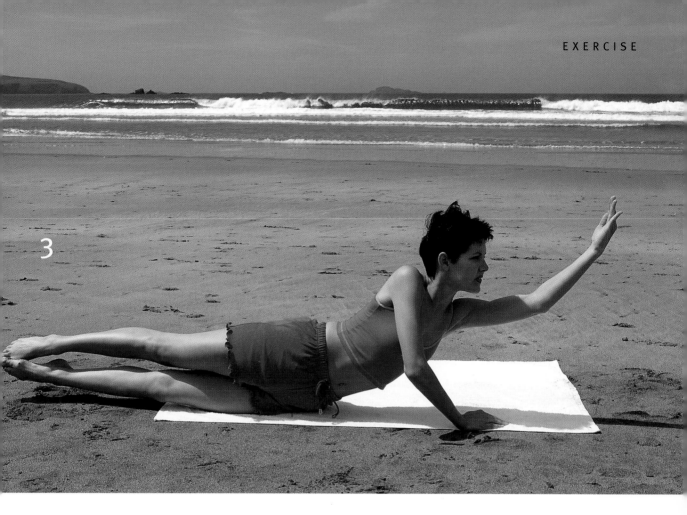

3

feet to feel as if you are in one straight line from the tips of your fingers to the tips of your toes. Place your upper hand on the floor for balance. Slowly raise both legs at once, keeping them together. Lower and repeat 8 times.

2 Now raise the upper body in a smooth, low curve, arm outstretched. Lower and repeat 8 times.

3 Finally, lift your legs and your upper body and then lower them again 8 times.

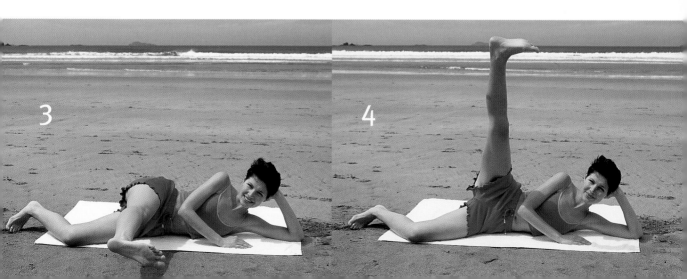

3

4

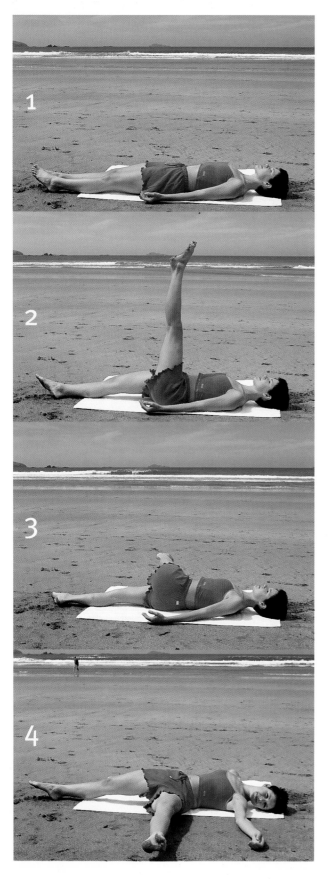

LEG SWEEPS

1 Lie flat on the floor on your back, with your knees and toes stretched and your stomach pressing back towards your spine.

2 Slowly lift your left leg straight upwards and then down towards your chest as far as it will go, keeping it straight.

3 Now let it cross the body and allow the weight of the leg to pull it down towards the floor.

4 Return the leg across the body and down to the floor in a smooth circle. Alternating legs, repeat 4 times on each side.

LEG KICKS

1 Lie flat on the floor on your back, with your knees and toes stretched and your stomach pressing back towards your spine. Lift your left leg, placing it so that it crosses over the right at the ankle.

2 Lift it again very slightly and let it drop down on the right ankle to bounce straight upwards. Lower and place the right leg on top, bounce and kick. Repeat for 8 kicks on each leg, keeping the movement smooth and elongated and the small of the back on the floor.

1

2

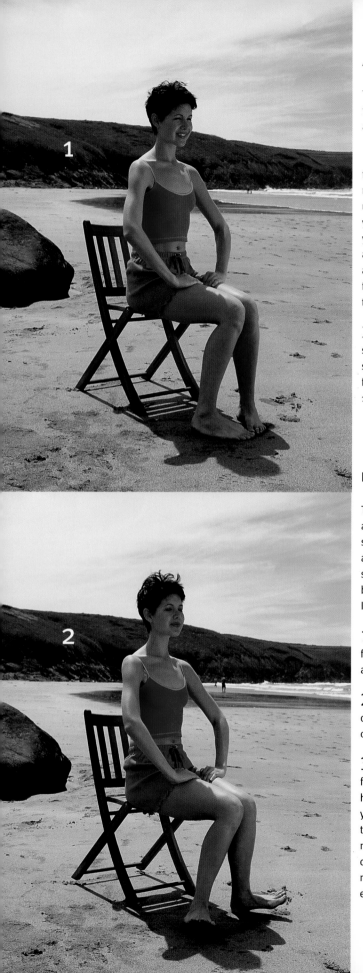

ANKLE TRIMMER

This is a wonderful exercise for shaping both the calves and the ankles.

1 Sit on the edge of a chair, feet flat on the floor, hands resting on your thighs, upper body relaxed. Keep your knees together but take your heels out so that they are about 15 cm (6 inches) apart, still resting on the floor. Keep your toes together.

2 Now sweep the toes out so that they make a little semi-circle, coming off the floor. Sweep in and out 16 times.

DOUBLE LEG STRETCH

This exercise could have just as easily appeared as a stomach strengthener. It is another Pilates-based sequence and one of the best all-round exercises that I know.

1 Lie on your back on the floor, legs outstretched and arms by your sides.

2 Raise your knees to your chest and rest your hands on your knees.

3 Keeping your stomach firmly held in, curve up your head and shoulders towards your knees, but without tensing up your shoulders or neck. Keeping the same curve in your back, pull your navel into your spine and extend your arms and legs so they are both pointing straight upwards.

4 In this position, turn out your legs from the hips and flex your feet (the more you flex, the better the exercise is for the thighs).

5 Keeping the feet and legs as they are, take your arms back towards your ears in the widest circle you can, up over your head and back to their previous position, stretching upwards.

6 When they are back to their starting point, point your toes and really stretch both arms and legs upwards. Bring your knees down to your chest and roll your back and head down to the floor. Work up to repeating this exercise 10 times.

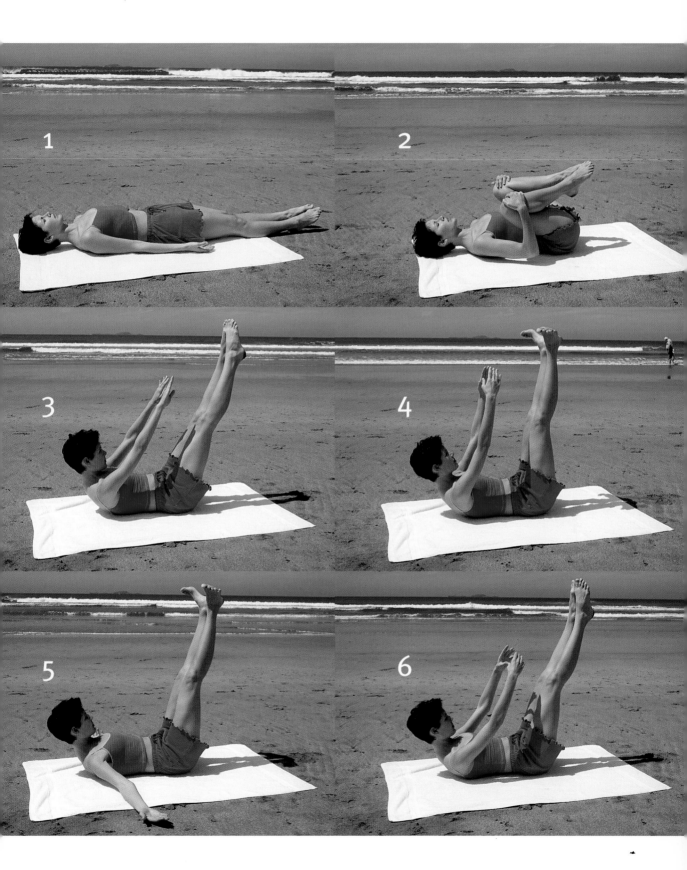

head and shoulders above the rest!

The exercises in this section are designed to remove tension in the neck and shoulders, improve posture and address particular problems such as flabby arms. Never let your shoulders hunch in tension or your spine slump; keep in front of you a mental picture of a lifted, elongated spine, a long neck and a gracefully held head. There will be an instant improvement in how you look.

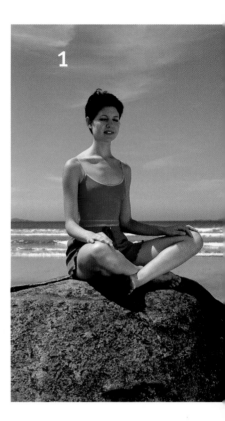

HEAD ROLLS

1 Standing or sitting with a straight spine and dropped, relaxed shoulders, let your head fall forwards onto your chest.

2 & 3 Very slowly, roll it around to the left until it is parallel with your shoulder – make sure you don't draw your shoulder up to meet it. Return to the centre and repeat on the right. Repeat the whole exercise 6 times.

SHOULDER LIFTS

1 Sitting or standing with a straight spine and a long neck, feel your shoulders dropped right down into your back.

2 Now lift them as high as you can – right up to your ears – then let them drop down. Repeat 8 times.

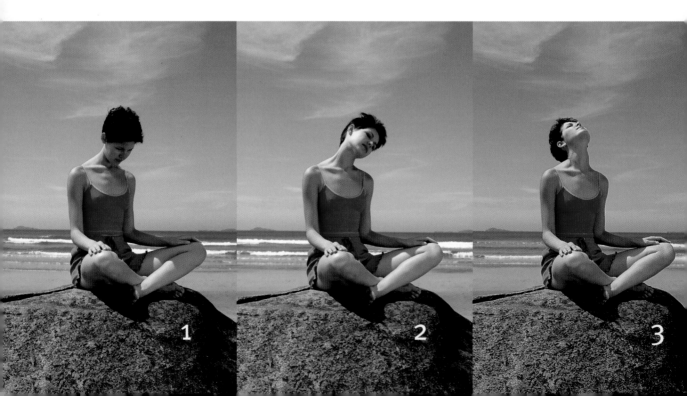

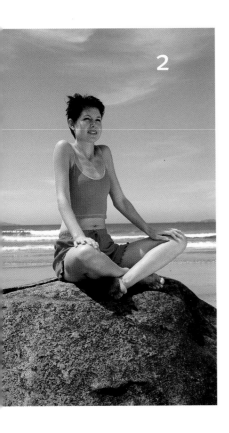

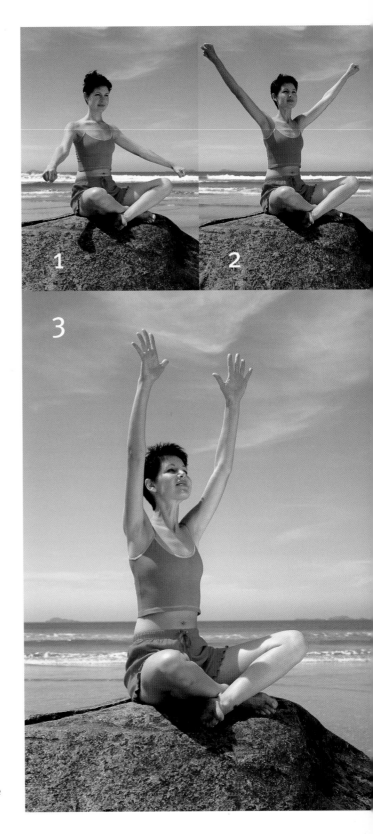

CLENCHING FISTS

1, 2 & 3 Sit cross-legged (or however you are most comfortable) with a straight back. Feel your body lifting up out of your waist and stretch your arms out low at your sides. Clench your hands into fists and then fling your fingers out, stretching them as far as they will go. Repeat the clenching and stretching as you raise your arms, taking 8 flings to get your arms pointing straight up and another 8 to get back down again. Build up to doing the whole exercise 4 times.

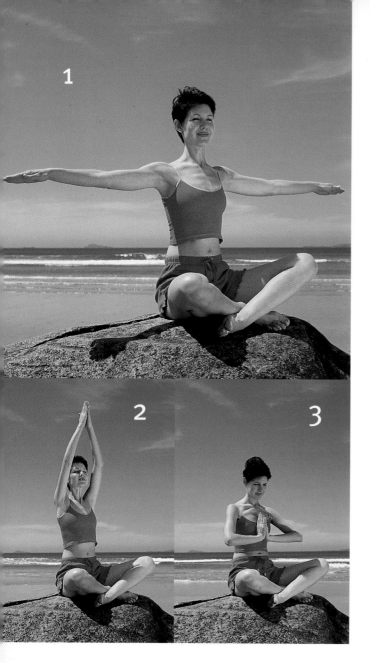

ARM CROSSES

This works on both the upper arms and the pectoral muscles.

1 Sit cross-legged with your arms stretched out in front of you, crossed at the wrist and pointing towards the floor.

2 & 3 From here, start to raise the arms, crossing and recrossing them, alternating which arm is on top. Take 8 crosses to reach the top and another 8 to come back down. Make sure you look straight ahead and keep your neck long. Repeat 4 times.

FLIPPER HANDS

This exercise is a really effective assault on flabby upper arms!

1 Sit cross-legged with your arms straight out to the side at shoulder level. Push away from the shoulders so that the arms are fully extended and flex the hands back, keeping the fingers straight so that you feel a stretch right along the underside of the arm.

2 Now drop the hands and curl them under as far as they will go. This time, you should feel a real pull along the backs of the hands, wrists and forearms. Repeat the sequence 16 times, keeping the shoulders dropped throughout.

BOSOM FIRMER

This works on the pectoral muscles that lie beneath the breast tissue – the breasts themselves have no muscles.

1 Sit cross-legged with your arms stretched out to the sides at shoulder level.

2 Raise your arms above your head until your palms meet, making sure your shoulders are dropped. Start to lower your hands in front of you, pressing them hard together as you do so. You should feel the pectorals working straight away, feeling almost as if they are pulling the arms down.

3 Lower your arms until your hands are in front of your breastbone, then take them out to the sides and repeat the whole sequence 4–8 times.

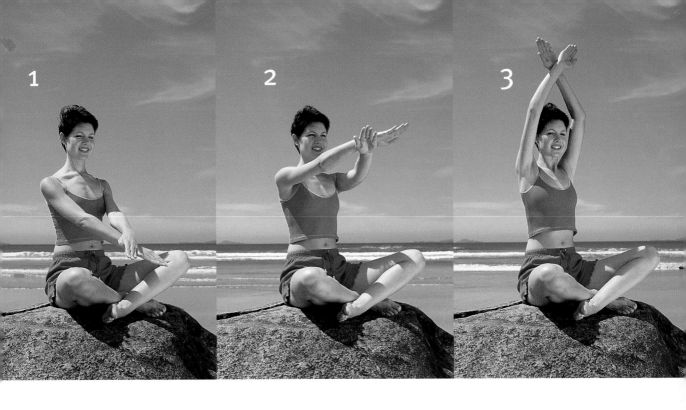

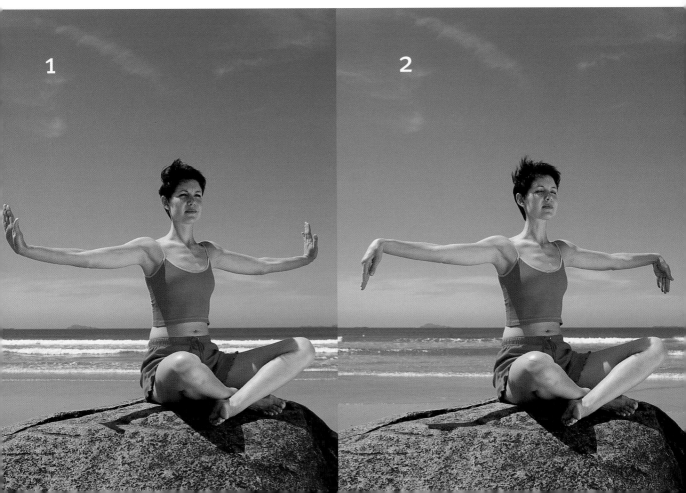

winding down

The end of an exercise session is just as important as the beginning. This is when the muscles are fully warmed up and can be stretched out, and when you should feel both relaxed and energized. Besides the exercises given here, you can also use any of the stretches on pages 18–27 and the roll down on page 14. You should find that your roll down is much more flexible by the end of a session and that your body feels generally looser. Any stiffness will disappear once you begin to exercise regularly.

ARM RELEASE

1 Sitting comfortably back on your heels or with crossed legs, raise one arm in the air.

2 Now fold it at the elbow so that your hand drops down towards the back of your neck.

3 With your other hand, push the raised elbow back and feel your hand drop further down your back. This is a gentle release – don't push too hard. Repeat on the other side.

REVITALIZING STRETCH

A revitalizing stretch will leave you feeling full of energy at the end of the exercise session.

1 Stand up straight, feet hip-width apart. Feel all your muscles pulled up.

2 Now let your breath out and, as you breathe in again, let the air fill your body and lift your arms out gently to the side. Breathe out as you lower them.

3 With each breath, lift the arms a little higher until they touch above your head. On the final intake of breath in the sequence, look up into your palms and bring the arms down again. The whole sequence should take around 8 breaths.

Now breathe normally for a few moments and feel your spine straight, your knees, thighs and stomach muscles pulled up, and your shoulders dropped down into the back and relaxed. Your head is lifted and in line with your spine. You should now feel full of oxygen and ready for anything!

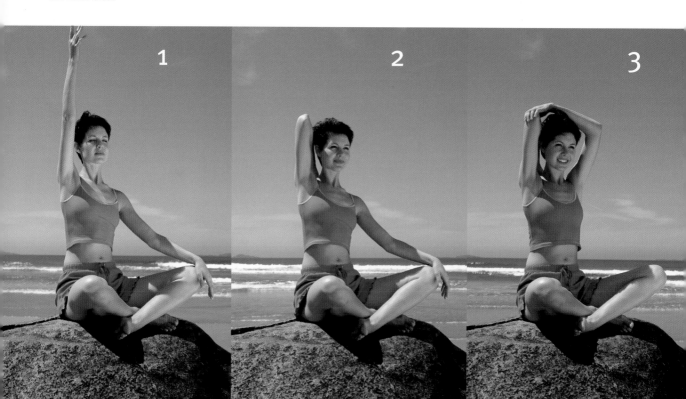

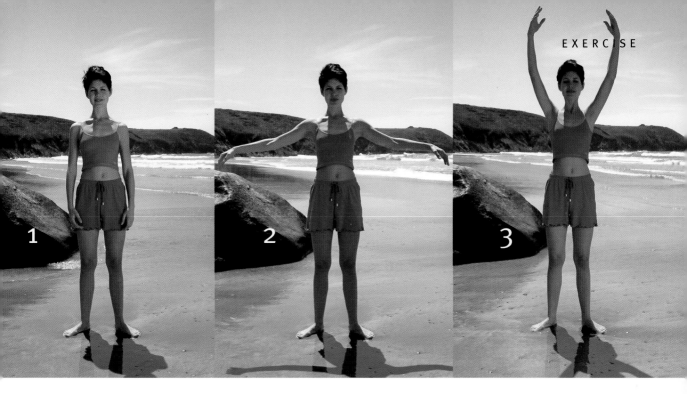

CHILD POSE

This is a traditional yoga
pose that is good for both
stretching and relaxing at
the end of a session.

1 Kneel down on the floor
and stretch your arms out in
front of you, feeling a long
pull the whole length of the
spine. Hold the stretch for
2 minutes.

2 Take one arm back and
lay it down at your side. (You
may want to move your head
at this point so that your
cheek is next to the floor if
this is more comfortable.)

3 Now take the second arm
back and lay it also down at
your side. Stay in this
relaxed pose for 2 minutes
or more and then get up
very slowly.

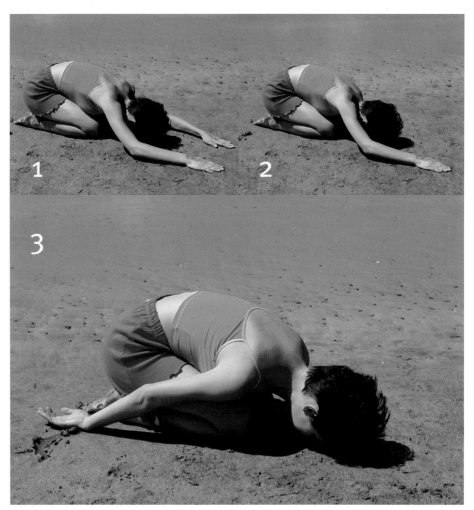

aerobic exercise

All of the exercises on the previous pages were for body toning and shaping. While these are excellent for defining and sculpting your figure, you do also need to do aerobic exercise. This does not necessarily mean 'aerobics' – there are plenty of other forms of aerobic exercise, such as swimming, cycling and running. However, aerobic exercise of some sort is vital for several reasons. First, and most importantly, it increases cardiovascular fitness. This means your heart muscle actually becomes stronger and pumps the blood around your body more efficiently. Aerobic exercise also protects against certain diseases – including coronary heart disease and, it is now thought, some types of cancer – and increases the mineral content of your bones, making problems such as osteoporosis less likely. It gives more flexibility to the joints, preventing stiffness and lack of mobility, and burns fat while building muscle.

Aerobic options

You don't have to do aerobic dance classes, but you can try them out to see if they suit you. Many people find the discipline of going to a class to exercise helps them to stick to it, and there is also the advantage of drawing support from the other people exercising along with you. If this doesn't appeal to you, though, there are plenty of other choices.

Walking

This is one of the easiest and best ways to exercise aerobically, but you do need to walk at a pace that will have an effect. Walk briskly with a long stride and breathe deeply. Wear sensible shoes and work right through the foot with each step – from heel to toe – to exercise the leg muscles and increase your speed as you get fitter. Try to do this for 20 minutes every day. The great advantage about walking as exercise is that you do not have to set aside a special time – you can do this on your way to work or to the shops.

Jogging

Although jogging is very popular and will certainly raise the heart rate, it does bring with it the possibility of damage to the joints – especially the knees – because of the impact of running on a street surface. If you enjoy jogging, try doing it on grass or on a treadmill in the gym and always wear good-quality supportive trainers. Three times a week for 20–30 minutes is ideal.

Swimming

This is one of the best forms of aerobic exercise, because with your body supported in water the chances of injuring yourself because of stress on the joints is virtually nil. Again, 20–30 minutes three times a week is ideal. There are also aquaerobics classes in many swimming pools now and these are good ways of exercising, too, as working against the water increases resistance and makes you work harder.

Cycling

Riding a bicycle is another excellent form of aerobic exercise – try cycling to work instead of getting the bus or go cycling with a friend at weekends. As with all aerobic exercise, little and often is best (20–30 minutes three times a week), building up speed gradually.

Other activities

Only those sports with a prolonged period where the heart rate is increased make good aerobic exercise – short spurts of activity don't count since the increase in the metabolic rate is not sustained. Consequently, the best sports for aerobics are enduring ones such as rowing. Dancing (provided it is non-stop) is good, too, as are activities such as skipping or trampolining.

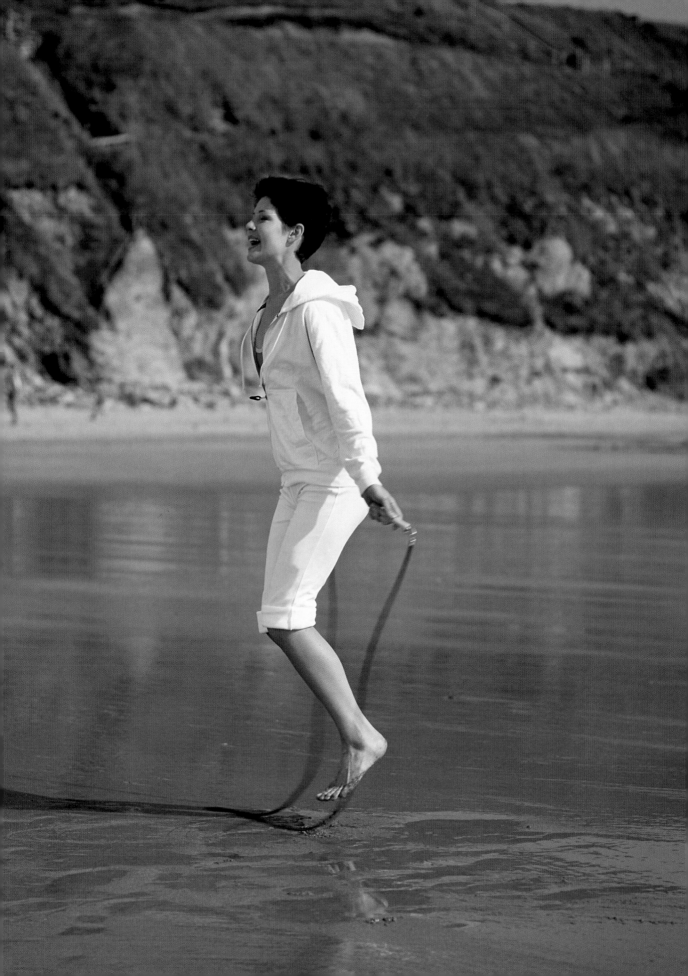

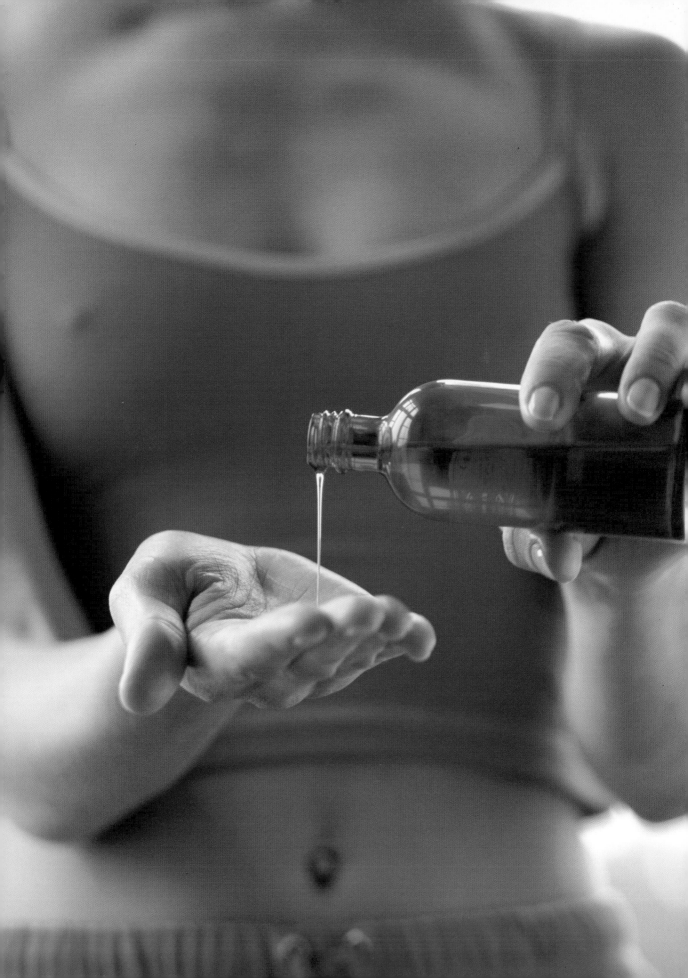

techniques and treatments

There are a number of techniques and treatments that will help increase the effectiveness of the 28-Day Vitality Plan. You can intensify the cleansing process with a number of detoxing techniques, some of which are real treats, too! Many of these, such as massage, saunas and steam baths, are widely available; there are also techniques you can do at home on a daily basis.

On the Plan, you start to feel better about yourself very early on because of the obvious improvements in your health and looks. However, this can be even further enhanced by making this a time to get rid of stress and to relax and calm your mind. And, because mind and body are so interlinked, the techniques described here for meditation and relaxation will also affect your physical health and well-being.

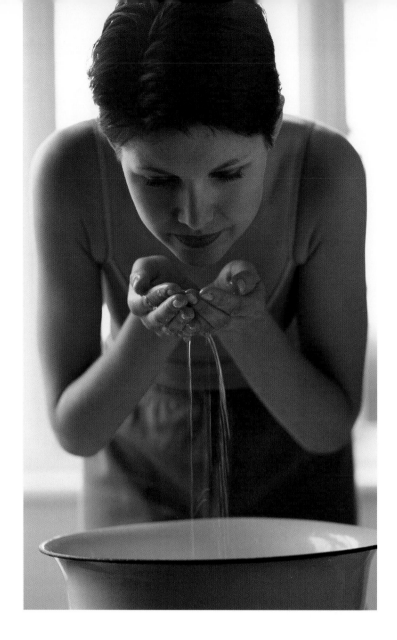

water treatments

Water is an important part of the 28-Day Vitality Plan. Not only do you drink lots of it, you can use hydrotherapy to speed up the cleansing process from the outside, too. Hydrotherapy is one of the oldest of the natural therapies and is extremely popular in the spas of Germany, Austria, Switzerland, Italy and France. Because it uses alternating hot and cold water, the effect on your system is extremely stimulating! In particular, it stimulates the circulation of the blood and the nervous system, but it is also believed to strengthen the immune system and encourage the elimination of toxins.

Morning shower routine
This may sound a bit scary but it's really worth doing – you'll find it has a remarkable effect on your whole system and gives you lots of energy to face the day. Start with skin brushing. For this you will need a natural bristle brush. You can get these

either with a detachable handle or with webbing and loops for handles, the latter being particularly good for brushing your back. Starting with the soles of your feet and using firm, long strokes, brush the whole of your body surface (not the face), moving upwards always towards the heart. On the abdomen, the movement is circular, in a clockwise direction. Be very gentle on the breasts and neck.

You will need to start skin brushing with a light pressure until you are accustomed to the feeling, then you can bring a slightly firmer pressure to bear. This is a very cleansing, stimulating and detoxifying technique and has the added benefit of making your skin beautifully smooth.

After skin brushing, your skin should be warm and tingling. Now for the hydrotherapy shower! Make sure the water is as hot as you can comfortably cope with and warm up your whole body with the water for 1 minute. Now turn the water to cold and let it flow over you for 30 seconds. Turn back to hot and repeat the whole process until you have had three hot and three cold showers, ending with the cold. Wrap yourself up in a warm towel and lie down for 5 minutes. You will find your whole body tingling with vitality – and your energy store will be increased throughout the day.

In the long term, these showers strengthen your immune system so you're less susceptible to every passing infection. Their supporters say they are even an anti-ageing tonic!

Water treats

There are a number of water treats you can give yourself either at home or at your local sports centre. Many sports centres now have saunas and these are a treat for detoxers. The ideal way of taking a sauna is in short bursts interspersed with a cold shower or a swim. Go in the sauna for 5–10 minutes at a time, then shower and rest for 5 minutes or swim before returning. Do this 3–4 times and then lie down quietly for 30 minutes – you should feel completely invigorated. Steam baths are also excellent and many people find their heat gentler than the dry heat of the sauna. In both, try to wear as little as possible and make sure you rest afterwards. Don't use either if you feel unwell or during the days of the actual juice fast itself.

There are also a number of baths you can take at home which are relaxing, stimulating or cleansing. One of my favourites is Moor mud, which comes from the Neydharting Moor in Austria and has been used for over 1000 years by everyone from Paracelsus, the 15th-century physician who called it 'the elixir of life', to Louis XIV and Napoleon and Josephine. While its modern-day adherents do not make quite such claims for Moor mud as Paracelsus did, they do believe it detoxifies and strengthens the whole system. It is particularly good if, during detox – or indeed at any other time – you suffer from skin complaints or from rheumatism or arthritis. Use Moor mud in the bath and soak before bedtime for at least 20 minutes. Pat yourself dry afterwards, wrap up warm and go straight to bed. There are other Moor products, too, including body lotion and oil and even a drink.

Dead Sea Mud is better known and has also been around for a long time. Cleopatra is said to have prized it so highly as a beauty treatment that she persuaded Mark Antony to conquer the region and present it to her as a gift. It contains an extraordinary range of minerals – especially large quantities of potassium – that help to regulate the body's water balance. It is also a relaxing bath and is thought to promote cell renewal and detoxing. As well as these general properties, it is recommended in particular for people with oedema, skin problems, sports injuries, rheumatism and arthritis.

Aromatherapy baths

Aromatherapy baths are wonderfully relaxing at the end of the day. Again, you should give yourself at least 20 minutes to absorb the oils and try to make your surroundings as relaxing as possible, too. Light a candle instead of turning the light on and listen to soft music. For a relaxing bath at the end of the day, try 5–10 drops of one or two of the following, mixed in well with the water before you get in:

- Lavender is one of the gentlest oils. It is safe to use directly on the skin, even with children. It has strong calming and sedative qualities and so is very effective for problems such as insomnia or any sort of tension. You can also put a few drops on your pillow to ensure a good night's sleep.
- Rose is a lovely scent which both relaxes and, it is said, rejuvenates. It is also very helpful with detox side-effects such as headache.
- Sandalwood is both calming and anti-depressant, so use it if you are feeling low and this is causing sleeplessness. It is of particular benefit to dry skin and has a lovely, woody, warm fragrance.
- Neroli is made from orange blossom and has a delicious, heady, floral scent. It is very uplifting as well as calming. It particularly suits dry or mature skin.

finding relaxation

During the plan, the aim is not just to detox the body but to detox the mind as well. This may seem a rather strange idea – after all, it is the body that tries to digest the wrong food, breathes in polluted air or suffers the side-effects of anti-biotics. However, stress can be regarded as the mind's toxin and this in turn has the effect not only of making us anxious, depressed or insomniac, it releases toxins into the body, too.

Just as the body affects the mind, the mind can affect the body. Noradrenalin, or norepinephrine, the neurotransmitter that is released during exercise, has the effect of lifting mood, while the effect of stress is to release adrenalin and this in turn puts the body under actual physical pressure. Our bodies have not fundamentally changed since prehistoric times when, as hunters, we would be exposed to extreme short-term dangers, such as being attacked by animals. In these situations, the body needed adrenalin to prepare it to fight the danger or to flee from it. However, while adrenalin is highly effective in helping us escape from short-term danger, it is not at all beneficial faced with the on-going, long-term stress that most of us have to cope with nowadays. In fact, adrenalin and the other chemicals our bodies produce in reaction to stress cause the body to produce its own toxic substances, the free radicals (see page 31). As we have seen, free radicals are impli-cated in the majority of human diseases, including cancer, heart disease, Alzheimer's disease and inflammatory and degenerative diseases.

That occurs, of course, in the long term but the immediate chemical effect of stress is to reduce the immune system's ability to function properly, thus making you more susceptible to disease. If stress is sustained over a prolonged period and develops into depression, corticosteroid levels are also raised and these put further pressure on the immune system. There is a growing body of research to link depression with an inability to fight cancer.

Stress relief

Clearly, we need to combat stress not only for our mental well-being, but for our bodies' well-being, too. There are a number of techniques that will relieve stress in a remarkably effective way. They include physical treatments from a therapist and long-term, daily practices that allow you to soothe your mind and be in control of your emotions rather than letting them control you.

Relaxation techniques

Even 10 minutes of relaxation a day will make a very big differ-ence to your stress levels, your ability to cope and your overall health. The following exercise is a relaxation used in yoga – you lie on the floor in what is known as 'the corpse position'. If you do this after a few sequences of Salute to the Sun (see page 24), you will find it of great benefit. Many people also find it helpful to record the following instructions on tape and play it while they do the relaxation. If you do this, ensure you speak very slowly, repeating each instruction several times if you like, and perhaps record some tranquil music in the background.

Your body temperature will drop during relaxation, so make sure you have something to cover yourself with. A pair of socks is also a good idea, as the feet can feel cold. Make sure you will not be disturbed, which would stop the whole relax-ation in its tracks.

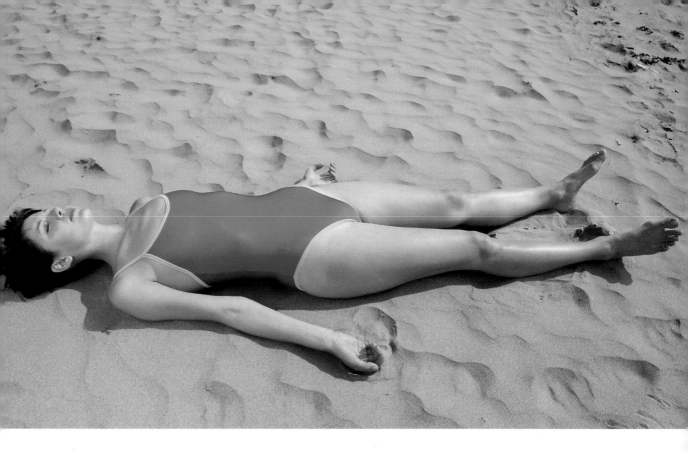

Lie on the floor with your feet about 45 cm (18 inches) apart, your legs rolling outwards slightly. Your arms should be straight but relaxed, your shoulders loose and your hands about 30 cm (12 inches) away from your body with the palms facing upwards. It may seem more comfortable to face the palms down, but when they are uppermost, the upper back and shoulders are more relaxed. Close your eyes. Make sure your shoulders are lowered and not tensed and your back is comfortably on the floor. Feel your whole body heavy on the floor.

Starting at your toes, begin to feel the relaxation spreading through your body, moving upwards like a wave. Spend time on each tiny part, putting all your concentration into each area of your body in turn, first the toes, then the feet and ankles. Feel the wave spreading up into your legs, through the shins and calves, the knees and into the thighs. Let your legs roll outwards from the hips. Let the hips and buttocks go – there is often a surprising amount of tension stored here. The whole body is softening and the effect now reaches the abdomen, which drops down further against the back, while the lower spine relaxes further into the floor.

The stomach, the waist and the ribs all expand and soften. The breathing is now probably quite light. As the softening, relaxing wave flows through the torso and into the back, they

fall deeper into the floor. The relaxation comes up into the shoulders and neck and out along the arms to the very ends of the fingers. The back of the neck is almost touching the floor, the scalp softens, almost loose against the skull, and the whole face – the jaw, the chin, the throat, the cheeks – melt away. The lips part and the tongue rests gently behind the lower teeth. The eyes sink gently back into the head and the temples and forehead smooth out.

The whole body is at rest. Enjoy this sensation, be aware of it. As thoughts come into your mind, watch them and see them float away like clouds in a summer sky. Any doubts or worries can float away in the same way as the physical tension has left your body. Stay in this place for 3–5 minutes. Now see the sun in your sky and feel its life-giving light and warmth. Feel the air around you and, as you take a deep breath in, feel that you are drinking in from the sun's vast source of energy, making you calmer and stronger.

Deepen the breath, letting the ribs expand and the lungs fill. After three breaths, begin to feel your toes and fingers coming to life. Wriggle them. Still with your eyes closed, lift your arms above your head and stretch your arms and legs away from each other. When you are ready, roll onto your side and open your eyes. Give yourself a few moments before you get up.

meditation

Meditation is not just daydreaming or relaxation; it works to train the conscious mind to a state of stillness and tranquillity and brings both physiological and psychological benefits. Many people feel that the Eastern or religious trappings associated with meditation mean that is not for them. In fact, meditation takes on many forms and philosophies and there is no religious bias necessary – you can take from it whatever it is you need. Primarily, it is a discipline for training your mind to a point of both deep concentration and relaxation.

Its early beginnings were, of course, religious, though it would be mistaken to imagine they were only Eastern – the early Christians meditated, too. The most common forms of

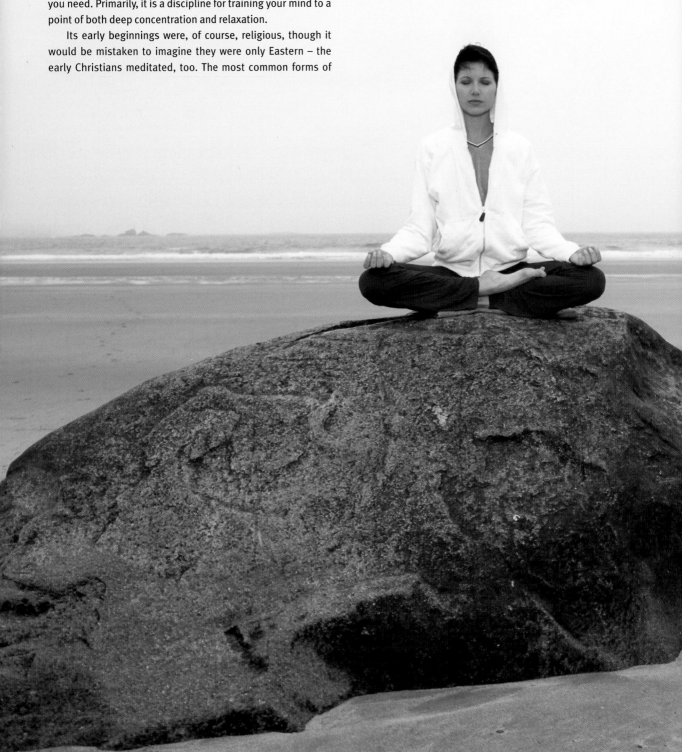

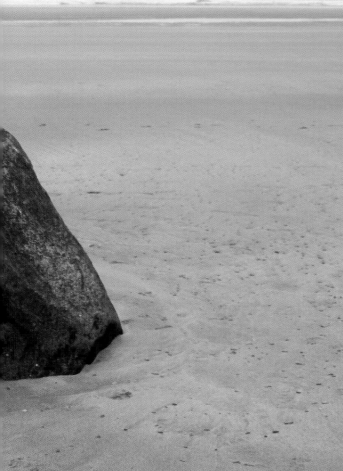

meditation we know today do come from the East and have been perfected over the centuries by such religions as Buddhism, Hinduism, Taoism and Islamic Sufism. Within this context, the aim of meditation is to help reach a point of spiritual enlightenment. However, for many people in the West today it is basically a practical self-help technique for coping with the high levels of stress found in our daily lives.

Methods of meditation may differ, but they all have in common the aim of producing a state of deep relaxation which, it is claimed, rejuvenates both mind and body. People who meditate regularly say it gives them a new zest for life, with increased energy, improved concentration and an inner peace that leads to better relationships. Sportsmen even claim it improves their performance.

When you see someone meditate, it looks as if very little is happening. You may notice that his or her breathing has slowed down, but otherwise he or she remains quite still, eyes closed. The work is all taking place on the inside. Most of the meditation techniques that are used these days are really concentration techniques. Their effect on the mind might be compared to the effect of exercise on the muscles of the body. They aim to tone up the capacity for memory, analysis, perception, inference, concentration, recognition and recall. By developing in these daily sessions the strength and flexibility of the mind, it is able to perform much more efficiently and effectively the rest of the time. In essence, it gives you the ability to stay focused on whatever you happen to be doing.

Learning to meditate

You can learn to meditate at home on your own simply by following the basic guidelines. There are numerous audio tapes available, too, to draw you through what is usually known as a 'guided meditation'. This may take the form of a journey or visualizing a series of images in your mind. There are also tapes that simply play 'meditational' music. However, unless you are meditating solely on that sound, these may prove to be more of a distraction than a help.

There have, of course, been many great teachers of meditation over the millennia. The most famous in our own century is the Maharishi Mahesh Yogi, who taught the Beatles and other pop stars to meditate and attracted countless Western devotees in the 1960s. He then went on to establish his Centres of Transcendental Meditation, which have now spread worldwide, using the technique of a repeated word or mantra. Many people do find it much more effective to have a teacher to guide them, especially when they are first starting to learn to meditate. Having other learners around can be helpful, too, making it easier to discuss difficulties.

The main thing to remember when learning to meditate is that the intrusion of thoughts is inevitable. Meditation is a technique it may take years to do with ease and this is only natural – you would not start learning tennis and expect to be playing at Wimbledon that week. Do not try too hard – you are not supposed to be forcing your mind into concentrating on a particular image. In fact, you are trying to release yourself from conscious thought. When anything enters your mind – thoughts, worries, ideas, lists of what you have to do when you stop meditating – observe its presence gently, make no judgement about the thought itself and, above all, do not become irritated with yourself for having it! Having recognized the thought, let it go, as if it floats away of its own accord, and draw your focus back to your breath, word or the image on which you are meditating.

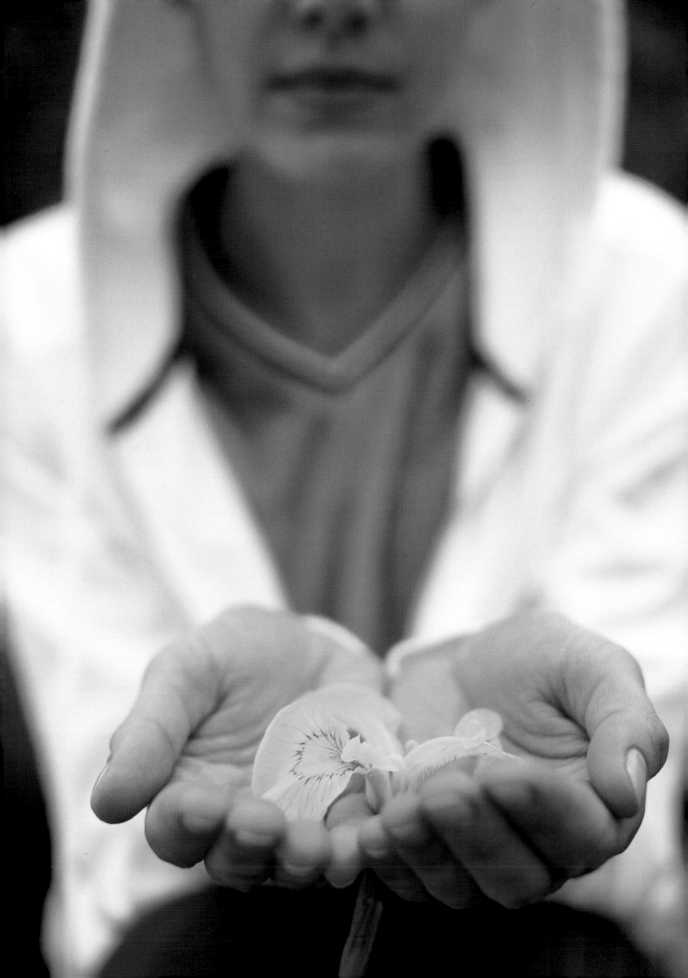

How meditation works

Nobody knows for sure how meditation works, though it can certainly be seen to quieten the mind and bring our thoughts under our control. In time, we become more able to control our thoughts and emotions in everyday life (not just when we are meditating) rather than being at the mercy of our emotions as so many people are. Most people who make a practice of meditating regularly find that they have greater clarity in all their thought processes, better memory and concentration and an ability to stay calm, by means of observing the thoughts and emotions that come into their minds and simply discarding those that will not be useful.

Clinical research has recorded a number of changes in the brain that take place during meditation. Electroencephalograph (EEG) tests show that electrical waves produced during meditation are different from those we produce at other times, whether asleep or awake. Electrical activity takes on a slow rhythm, with regular, even waves recorded from different parts of the brain. This evenness and regularity continue after meditation, too, with sustained practice.

This change in brain wave pattern is called alpha rhythm and is associated with feelings of peace and tranquillity. Commonly reported beneficial side-effects by meditators include reduced stress levels, improvement in insomnia and quality of sleep and a reduction in any tendency towards addiction (cigarettes, alcohol, drugs or food). Medical research since the 1960s has shown that meditation has marked physiological effects, many of which are beneficial for stress-related conditions. Specific effects include:

- Lowering the blood pressure
- Slowing the pulse rate
- Slowing the respiratory rate, but with the same levels of oxygen in the blood
- Reduction of activity of the autonomic nervous system
- Improvement in circulation
- Reduction of harmful lactic acid in the body.

Research is still going on into whether meditation can have any effect on cancer. Certain types of cancer are thought to appear at times of great stress because stress can damage the function of the immune system, which is needed to destroy cancer cells. Diminishing stress by meditation is therefore thought by some practitioners to have a place in cancer treatment though, as yet, there has not been sufficient research to judge.

Preparing for meditation

Meditation is not complicated, but it does require regular practice if it is to be of benefit. Start with one, or preferably two, 10-minute sessions a day and build up to 20 minutes for each. You need to be comfortable but alert to meditate. Do not try to meditate while you are very tired – you will probably just fall asleep – or when you have recently eaten or drunk alcohol. You should also avoid being disturbed – take the phone off the hook, if necessary. Find a quiet spot, wear loose, comfortable clothing and take off your shoes.

You do not have to sit in a yogic posture to meditate, though if you are used to a lotus or half-lotus they can be a very comfortable way of holding a position for 20 minutes. You can sit cross-legged on the floor or in a straight-backed chair. However, it is important to be able to sit with a straight back and stay still for the session, so choose something you know your body can take without strain.

Before you begin, take a few moments to focus on your body. Take some slow, deep breaths and try to let go of any areas of tension. Finally, scan your mind for immediate thoughts and worries. Observe them and simply leave them on one side for later so your mind is clear to meditate.

Meditation techniques

It does not really matter which meditation technique you use. Generally, people find that one suits them better than another. However, it is important to give each one a try – say, 10 days before you decide whether to try another. When you have found a method you like, the most important thing is to practise it regularly. Try to make your meditation session the same time of day in the same place. When you become adept, you will be able to meditate at any time and in all kinds of places – even when there is noise or other people around.

Breathing meditations There are several different forms. Start with the easiest, which is to count each breath. Inhale on one, exhale on two, inhale on three and so on. The breath should be even and you can focus the counting on either the sensation of the air entering through the nose or the rise and fall of the abdomen. If you lose count, start again at one. The second form of counted breathing counts only the exhalations – this is harder because the gaps between counting are longer. Finally, count the inhalations. On the inbreath, the mind is inclined to wander more easily, making this slightly more difficult again. Finally, simply follow the breath without counting. Observe the natural flow of your breath, the movement of the abdomen, as you would watch the gentle breath of a sleeping child.

Focusing This form of meditation can again take many different forms. A good way of starting is to close your eyes and become aware of your own physical body lying on the floor or sitting on the chair and the everyday noises around you, such as cars going by, dogs barking, babies crying. Simply observe them and then let them go. A more concentrated form is to focus upon a particular object. This may be anything small and static – perhaps a flower, a stone or a candle flame – which should be placed in front of you, preferably about 90 cm (3 feet)

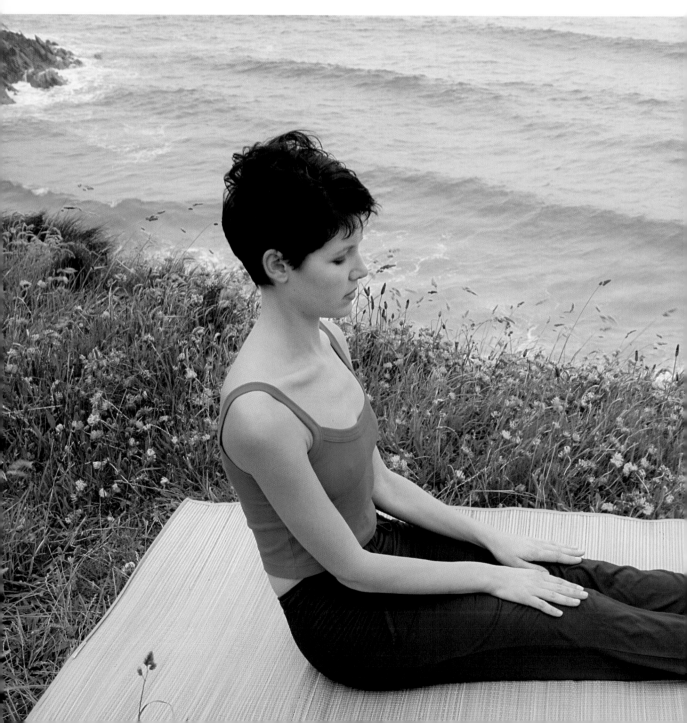

away and at your eye level. Look, without blinking, at the object for a minute, or as long as you can. Then close your eyes and look at the imprint it has left in your mind's eye. When the image fades, open your eyes and look again, alternating in this way to the end of the session.

Colour Choose any colour and, closing your eyes, try to fill your mind with it to the exclusion of everything else. It may be helpful to start by giving the colour a picture – a green field, a blue sky or a yellow sun. Then gradually try to go in closer so that you can no longer see the outlines of your picture and the colour floods your mind.

Mantra A mantra can be any word repeated aloud or silently on which the mind focuses. It can be a word with significance for you, like 'peace', or one that has a resonant sound – the best-known being the 'Om' mantra (pronounced 'aum'). Your aim is to reach a stage where the sound and resonance fill your mind.

Visualization This can take the form of a place or an object, real or imagined, that you look at with your mind's eye. You picture this in the greatest detail, focusing completely upon it. Visualizing a place of great tranquillity has a particularly calming influence in this meditation.

After meditation
After 10–20 minutes, allow the focus of your meditation to fade gently away and bring your mind back to the present. Take some long, deep breaths and let your focus take in your body and how it is feeling, gradually becoming aware of your surroundings and the noises around you. Open your eyes and do a little gentle stretching. You are now refreshed for the rest of the day.

Remember, meditation can seem quite difficult to many people because their minds are full of thoughts and apparently unable to focus for any time at all on any of the techniques. This is quite normal. Do not feel that you are 'failing' to meditate; it is all part of the process of stilling the mind. If you try one of the above methods and find it does not suit you, try another. In any case, with time and practice, the ability to quieten the mind improves and these thoughts will bother you less.

Spiritual meditation
Many people who meditate find not only a sense of deep personal inner peace, but also of connectedness with those around them and of an inner store of wisdom and strength which is available to them to tap into whenever they need it. This often encourages them to explore the more spiritual and religious aspects of meditation. There are many Buddhist centres around for those who are interested, as well as a wealth of books on such subjects. More advanced methods of meditation should certainly be learned under the guidance of an experienced teacher and will inevitably have a moral and spiritual element, though not necessarily a religious one.

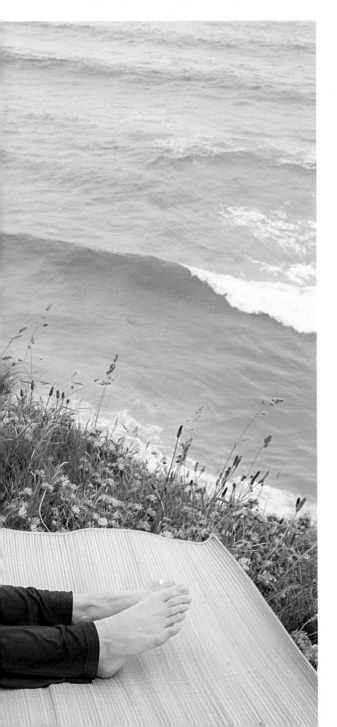

massage

Massage is one of the most delightful treatments we can experience. When done well, it can be deeply relaxing for both body and mind. When you are on the 28-Day Vitality Plan, the rougher strokes of conventional Swedish massage are probably not appropriate but there are many other forms that can be very effective. One of the most pleasant forms of massage is aromatherapy; the scents are in themselves both beneficial and uplifting, and the oils can help dry, damaged or problem skin. There are aromatherapists now in all parts of the country and some will even come to you, which is especially relaxing. You can go straight to bed if you have a massage in the evening and you will usually experience a perfect night's sleep.

If you are doing the Plan with a friend, you could give each other a regular aromatherapy massage. It is quite simple to learn to give a massage – there are plenty of books around to show you the strokes and, most importantly, you follow your own instinct and the reactions of the person who is being massaged. If she or he finds that one area is very tense and needs more attention or simply that a particular stroke feels good and brings a deeper relaxation, you can concentrate on that. Choose oils that have uplifting and relaxing qualities, such as lavender, rose, neroli, ylang-ylang, geranium, jasmine or the citrus oils and make sure you dilute them properly. For use on the body, dilute 25 drops of essential oil in 50 ml (2 fl oz) of carrier oil, such as almond, grapeseed or peach. Reduce the essential oil by half if you are going to use it on the face.

Lymphatic drainage

Lymphatic drainage is another kind of massage. It stimulates the lymphatic system and releases stored toxins for elimination. The lymphatic system is essentially your immune system. Lymph flows around the body, rather like the blood, except that it does not have the heart to pump it, relying instead on the normal contracting and relaxing of your muscles. Besides carrying various substances and chemicals around the body, the main function of the lymphatic system is to destroy bacteria and viruses and break down other toxins for elimination. The tonsils and adenoids have large amounts of lymphatic tissue, as do the spleen and liver. Exercise helps to stimulate the lymphatic system so that the wastes and toxins are eliminated regularly – which is obviously vital if your immune system is to work efficiently. In lymphatic drainage, the masseuse works directly on the lymphatic system to encourage it to throw off toxins more rapidly and improve its functioning generally. Besides the stimulation of the immune system, it is said to be of great benefit in removing cellulite. Contact your local sports centre or gym to find a practitioner.

Panchakarma

Massage is only a part of true *panchakarma*, which is itself only one element of the ancient Indian system of Ayurvedic health. When you embark on full *panchakarma* – the whole thing can take up to four weeks – it is a very cleansing and revitalizing experience, but on the 28-Day Vitality Plan the massages alone are very beneficial.

Abhyanga massage entails the use of warmed sesame oil, which is administered by two masseurs at the same time, working in tandem on both sides of the body. Sesame oil has been shown to contain antioxidants and to have anti-carcinogenic effects. *Abhyanga* massage stimulates the release of toxins from the cells and uses a quite different stroke from the forms of massage we are more used to. The strokes are mostly long and firm and those parts of the body not being massaged are covered in hot towels, heat being part of the cleansing process.

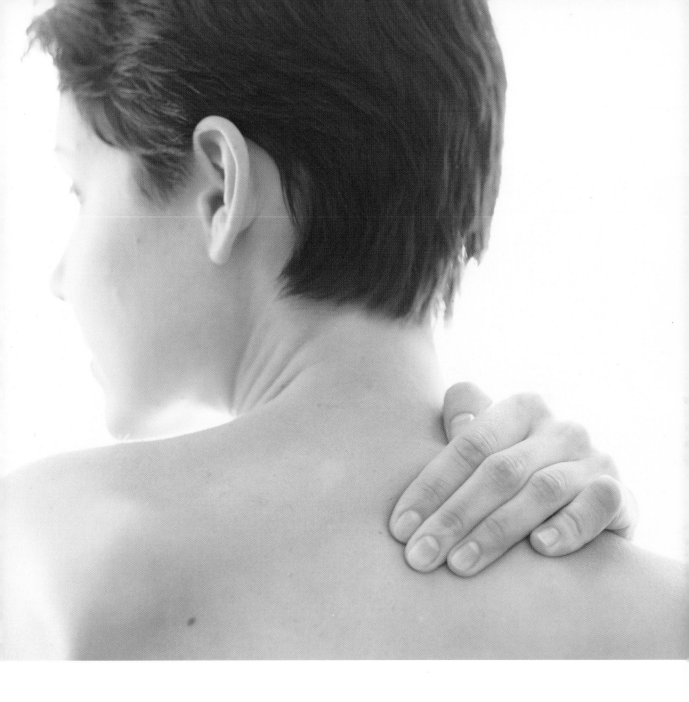

Herbs are also added to the hot sesame oil, chosen to suit your body/metabolism type (known in Ayurveda as *doshas*) and to remove imbalances in the body.

The second 'massage' can only be called a massage of the mind. In *shirodhara*, a stream of sesame oil is drizzled onto the forehead from a dish with a hole pierced in it. The oil begins on the centre of the forehead and moves slowly from side to side, pausing in the centre, for about 20 minutes in all. Most people find this profoundly relaxing and, according to Ayurveda, it strengthens the central nervous system. EEG tests have shown that brain wave coherence is enhanced after *shirodhara*.

There are several other forms of treatment you will experience if you decide to try full *panchakarma*. There have been various studies on its effects. One is on lipid peroxide levels, the damaged molecules that can deteriorate into free radicals when attacked by them. The results showed that levels temporarily went up as the system was stimulated by *panchakarma* and threw off the rogue molecules and then lowered very significantly. Other studies showed a marked decline in anxiety as measured by a standard psychological test and a rise in HDL (high density lipoprotein – the beneficial type of cholesterol) after *panchakarma*.

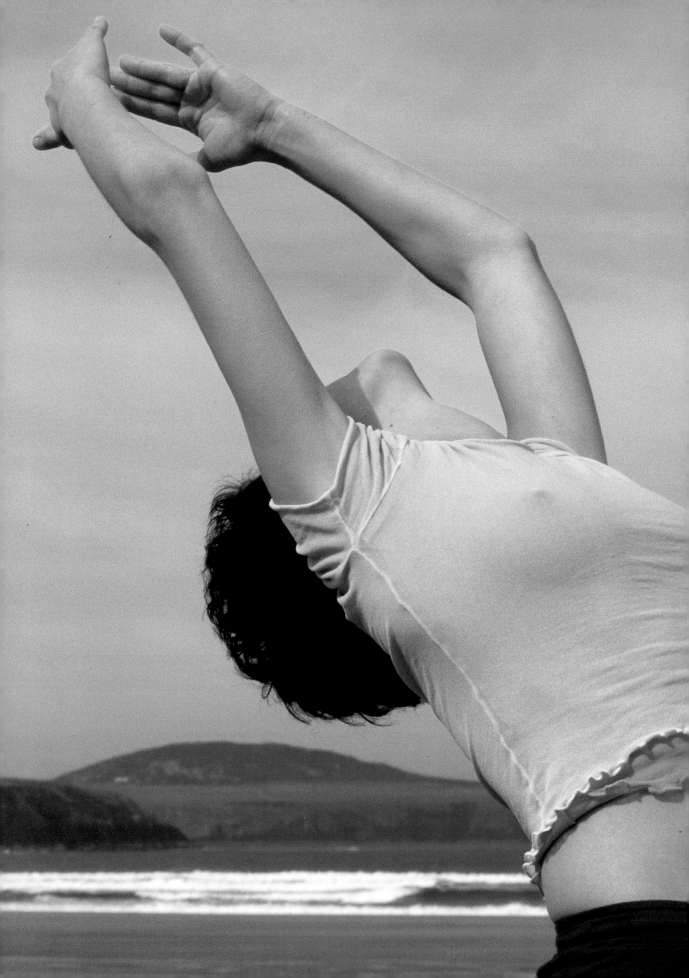

one-month make-over

This section of the book shows you how to put together the various elements of the 28-Day Vitality Plan – posture, exercise, diet, juicing – for its most effective use. This is not going to be the same for everyone. If, for instance, you are already fit and a regular exerciser, you will be able to do much more taxing exercise right from the start. This is not, though, a competition – don't push yourself into doing things before you're ready.

These are four weeks you have given to yourself as a time to concentrate on you. By the end of them (and probably quite a while before that) you will look and feel better and you will have given your body the chance to rest and renew. This is your time – enjoy it.

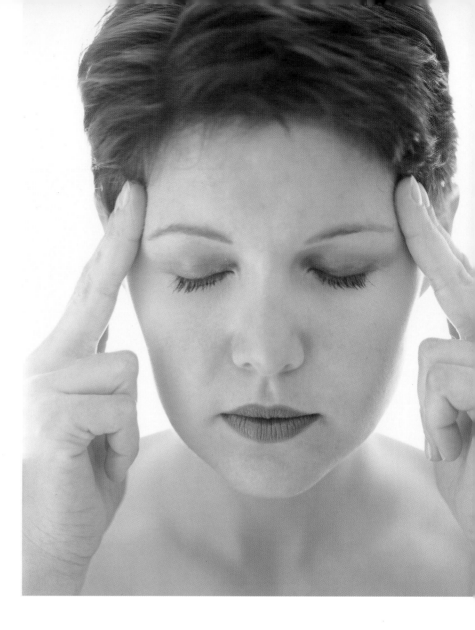

week one

This is your juice detox week, and for that reason it may seem the hardest. In fact, it isn't nearly so difficult as you might imagine, because the juices themselves are delicious and you wind down to them gradually. If you feel daunted by the idea of three days with only liquids, start with one or two and see how you feel. You can always break the fast or continue with it depending on how you feel. Bear in mind, though, that everyone has some sort of side-effect – it's nothing to panic about, it's just the toxins coming out.

The way you start and end the juice fast is very important. The week before you begin, eat as much salad and fruit as you can, try to steer clear of alcohol and very fatty or processed foods and get plenty of sleep. Make the effort to take some exercise and if you smoke cut right back now, because you can't smoke during the Plan itself – and afterwards you'll feel so much better you won't want to start again.

Even though you are drinking juices, you will still need to drink more fluids. Herb teas (not black tea) or filtered or bottled water are best.

Posture

Start with the deep breathing routine (see page 16) for 5 minutes every morning – if you like, you can even do it in bed before you get up. Do the roll down slowly every morning, too,

4–5 times (see page 14). Try to feel your body's alignment, with everything fitting neatly as you roll back up. Then choose some of the Pilates or stretches and do these for 10–15 minutes. The easiest ones to start with are the waist twists (see page 18) and the tennis ball (see page 20) from Pilates and, in the stretches, the back stretch (see page 21) and (if you work up to it gradually) Salute to the Sun (see page 24). Once more during the course of the day – either in the afternoon or last thing at night – do the breathing routine again.

Aerobic exercise

If you hardly exercise at all, start off slowly. Try to take a little aerobic exercise (see page 90) each day, perhaps just a brisk walk. This doesn't have to be a special journey. Why not get off the bus a stop or two early and walk the last bit? Then this can gradually be increased during the week. If you can, try to fit in one other aerobic session during the week – perhaps go for a swim or try out a gentle exercise class. If you're more accustomed to exercising, try to add in one extra session during the course of the week.

Body toning

At least two or three times this week, try to fit in 20 minutes for body toning. There is no doubt going to be one area in particular you want to concentrate on, but do at least one exercise from each section and always do the warm-up (see page 62). If you're starting from scratch, choose from those below. If you're already fitter than this, go on to the tougher ones from the second or third weeks, but don't push your body further than it is ready to go.

Trim torsos Stomach muscles need to strengthened gradually. Don't force your body to do something of which it isn't yet capable. If your stomach muscles start to bulge or quiver, stop immediately.
- Torso twists (see page 66)
- Side stretches (see page 66)
- Roll-ups (first and/or second versions) (see page 68)

Beautiful bottoms Always check your posture before you start. A sway in the back will mean not only that the exercise is not nearly as effective, it can damage your back, too.
- Buttock awareness (see page 71)
- Back leg lifts (see page 70)
- Turn-out (see page 74)
- Deep pliés (see page 75)

Thigh trimmers Skin-brushing (see page 94) will help, as well as specific exercises. Don't forget to stretch out the legs completely for maximum effect.
- Parallel pliés (see page 76)
- Leg lifts (first version) (see page 78)
- Inner thigh lifts (see page 77)
- Ankle trimmer (see page 82)

Head and shoulders Don't forget these exercises – they help to get rid of stored tension in the neck and shoulders as well as toning up your arms.
- Head rolls (see page 84)
- Shoulder lifts (see page 84)
- Bosom firmer (see page 86)

Winding down Always give yourself a few moments at the end of a session to stretch and get ready to go again.
- Roll down (2–3 times) (see page 14)
- Revitalizing stretch (see page 88)

Techniques and treatments

The most important techniques this week are those that will speed up the elimination process – skin brushing and the hydrotherapy shower (see page 94). It may sound a bit daunting at first but, after you've done it a few times, you'll find it exhilarating and energizing. Make sure you do it in a warm bathroom and wrap up in a warm towel afterwards. If the juice fast gives you headaches or makes you feel tired or tetchy, have an aromatherapy bath last thing at night with rose or lavender oil in it. It will help clear the headache and ensure a good night's rest.

It is also important this week to start a relaxation technique (see page 96) or meditation (see page 98) as these will actually help the detox programme, as well as calming the mind at a time when rest is very important. This should be kept up throughout the 28-Day Vitality Plan, as should the skin brushing and hydrotherapy.

Remember, this week is the one you build on for the whole Plan – so try to stick to it even if you find it quite hard going. You are also more likely to experience side-effects this week than you are from next week on. Try to continue with the detox even if you have a headache or other symptoms – though if you feel ill, you should, of course, see your doctor. If you find the juice fast difficult, go on to the post-fast regime, but keep that up for the rest of the week. And it is certainly true that the first day of juice-only is the hardest – each day gets easier after that!

week two

By the beginning of this week you should already be feeling much healthier, as well as having shed a few unnecessary pounds – just how many really depends on how long you continued the juice fast and how much you needed to lose. Even if you only did a one-day juice fast, though, you will be feeling noticeably more slender. This is not the point at which you rush to the refrigerator and eat everything in sight, though! You should come back slowly to a balanced diet – the point of last week, after all, was in part to re-educate your body to a healthy way of eating.

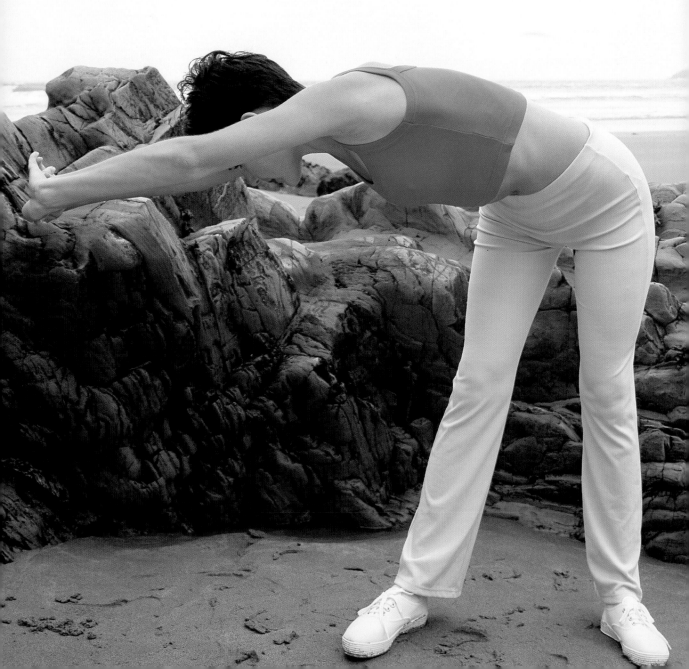

Diet

This week, you eat three meals a day again, but keep them light. If you become hungry in between – in fact, you probably won't – snack on fruit. Besides the juice at breakfast, have another one or two glasses of freshly made juice each day.

Breakfast Choose the lighter ones, such as Seedy Yogurt (see page 47) and Gingered Apples (see page 46), at least for the first half of the week. Have some freshly made juice and a cup of herb tea, too. If you're really haunted by the thought of coffee, try a herbal substitute.

Lunch and dinner This week, lunch and dinner should be soup or salad. Decide which you want at which time, but have one of each every day. You can take soup to work with you in a flask or put a salad in a container (but keep the dressing separate until you're ready to eat it). If you're making soup, don't forget to make extra and freeze some for another day. Choose from any of the soups (see pages 48–51) and from the following salads:
- Guacamole and Crudités (see page 52)
- Mushroom, Courgette and Tomato Salad (see page 52)
- Red Leaf Salad (see page 53)
- Bulgar Wheat Salad (see page 53)
- Cottage Garden Salad with Strawberries (see page 53)
- Continental Mixed Salad (see page 55)
- Mixed Leaf Salad with Spiced Nuts (see page 55)
- Celeriac Salad (see page 55)
- French Bean and Apricot Salad (see page 55)

Posture

Continue with the breathing routine (see page 16) and roll down (see page 14) and add the cat (see page 20). From the stretches, increase the number of sequences from Salute to the Sun (see page 24).

Aerobic exercise

Try to increase the amount of aerobic exercise you're taking – make sure you take a brisk walk daily at a time that fits in with your routine and make time for one or two 20-minute (or longer) sessions of other aerobic exercise, such as swimming, cycling or an exercise class.

Body toning

Do the warm-up (see page 62) and, if you're feeling stronger and more toned since last week, add some or all of the following to your toning regime:

Trim torsos
- If you feel comfortable with the side stretches (see page 66), go on to the upper body circles (see page 66). These call for a lot more strength in the abdominals, so don't overdo it – and if anything hurts, stop
- Do the first set of roll-ups (see page 68) and add the second. If you're feeling much stronger, try the third

Beautiful bottoms
- Leg circles (see page 72)
- Leg stretches (first sequence) (see page 72)
- Foot tapping (20 taps) (see page 74)

Thigh trimmers
- Leg sweeps (see page 80)
- Double leg lifts (first version) (see page 78)

Head and shoulders
- Clenching fists (see page 85)

Winding down
- Roll down (see page 14)
- Back stretch (see page 21)
- Last stretch (see page 88)

Techniques and treatments

Continue with the skin-brushing and hydrotherapy showers (see page 94), as well as the relaxation (see page 96) or meditation (see page 98). If you have found one form of meditation difficult, try another technique or, if you'd prefer to, go to a class to learn it.

This week, as you start to step up the aerobic exercise as well as the toning, you'll probably feel a few muscular aches and pains. If you do, a good way of relaxing is in a Moor or a Dead Sea mud bath. Give yourself plenty of time to soak before going to bed and don't dry yourself vigorously with the towel – just pat gently.

week three

This week you will see a big difference in how you look and feel. You will almost certainly be feeling more alert and positive about yourself and will have lost weight and be more toned. So perhaps now is a good idea to try an exercise class if you haven't so far. It's also time to give yourself a treat in recognition of what you've achieved so far (see Techniques and Treatments).

Diet
You can now choose from all the salads and all the soups – one of each a day as before – and any of the breakfasts. If you want, you can also substitute one of the following main meals for a soup or salad meal:
- Pasta with Three Herb Sauce (see page 58)
- Pasta with Tomato Sauce (see page 58)
- Vegetable Hot-Pot (see page 56)
- Stir-Fried Vegetables (see page 56)
- Steamed Vegetables with Ginger (see page 56)
- Baby Corn with Alfalfa (see page 56)
- Hot Scallop Salad (see page 57)
- Chinese Noodles and Prawns (see page 59)

Make sure you continue to drink at least 1.8 litres (3 pints) of water a day and make one or two fresh juices daily, too.

Posture
Always starting with the breathing routine (see page 16) and the roll-down (see page 14), you can now include any of the Pilates exercises and stretches – but stop if you feel under any strain. Make sure you stretch gently. Don't try to force your body into a position it can't reach, as this will only cause damage in the end. Remember to do the breathing routine again during the course of the day.

Aerobic exercise
You should now be working towards two or three 20-minute aerobic sessions per week, preferably fast walking, swimming, cycling, aerobic exercise classes, trampolining or skipping.

Body toning
Do the warm-up (see page 62) as usual. If your body is feeling comfortable with the exercises from last week, build on these gradually, adding or substituting from the following:

Trim torsos
- If you are able to do the first two stages of the roll-ups without straining, go on to the third (see page 68)
- Rope climbing (see page 69)
- Crossed fists (see page 69)

Beautiful bottoms
- Foot tapping (work up to 50 taps) (see page 74)

Thigh trimmers
- Leg kicks (see page 80)

Head and shoulders
- Arm crosses (see page 85)

Winding down
- Child's pose (see page 89)

Techniques and treatments
As well as continuing the hydrotherapy showers and skin brushing (see page 94) from the previous weeks, try to combine a swim with a session in a sauna or steam room. This will be wonderfully cleansing and invigorating and if you have an afternoon or an evening to spare you will find it very relaxing, too.

You should be finding that your stress levels are much more under control now if you have made meditation (see page 98) or relaxation techniques (see page 96) a part of your regular routine. Continue with these and, if you can, have a professional massage (see page 104) or, alternatively, take turns with a friend to give a massage to each other.

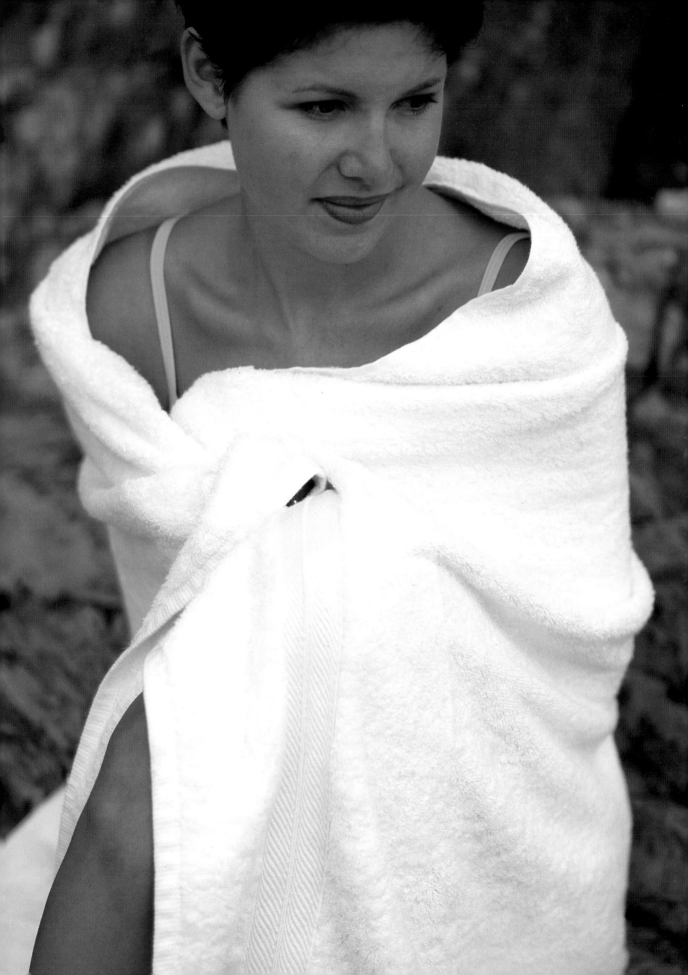

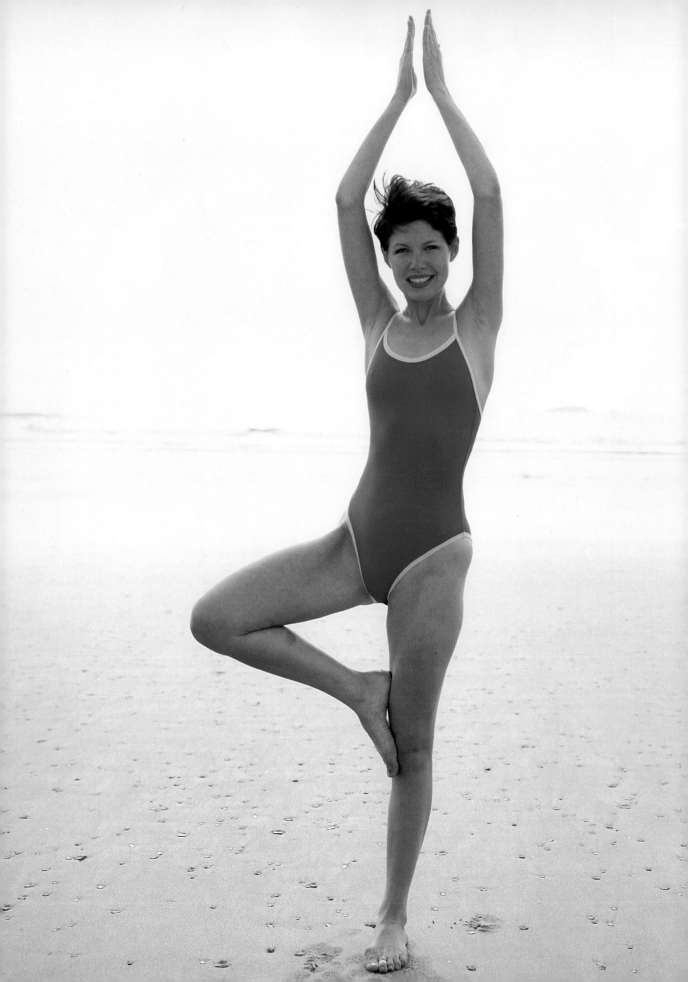

week four

This week is the final part of the 28-Day Vitality Plan and a time of consolidation and preparation for the future. If you've kept to the plan this far, you'll certainly be feeling and looking much better than when you started, as well as being much healthier on the inside, with a much-improved immune system. Give yourself a pat on the back – buy a new outfit or get a new haircut to suit the new you.

Diet

You can now choose from any of the options – breakfasts, soups, salads and main meals. However, try to ensure you have a high intake of the antioxidants and nutrients you need. Eat lots of salads and fresh fruit and keep on drinking plenty of filtered or bottled water. Drink at least one glass – preferably more – of freshly made juice each day.

Posture

Carry on with the breathing and posture routines as part of starting your day so that you begin with your body in alignment. You should be much more aware now of your posture – try to check it throughout the day to make sure that you sit, stand and walk in the best way.

Aerobic exercise

Keep building on this to a sensible level – there's no need to do more than three 20-minute sessions a week of intensive aerobic exercise, especially if you are doing plenty of walking and taking the stairs instead of the lift.

Body toning

You can now incorporate any of the exercises in this section, provided your body feels ready for them. Never push yourself beyond your present capabilities. If you take things at your own pace you'll progress, but if you try to force the pace you may well strain or injure yourself.

Techniques and treatments

Continue with the skin-brushing and hydrotherapy showers (see page 94), as well as the meditation (see page 98) and relaxation techniques (see page 96).

At this point, you may want to start investigating other techniques and treatments in more depth, for instance Pilates, Alexander Technique, yoga or the deep-cleansing therapy of *panchakarma*. You will also, no doubt, have found something extra you enjoy – maybe a sauna or a massage. Try to incorporate these into this week and the weeks to come if you can.

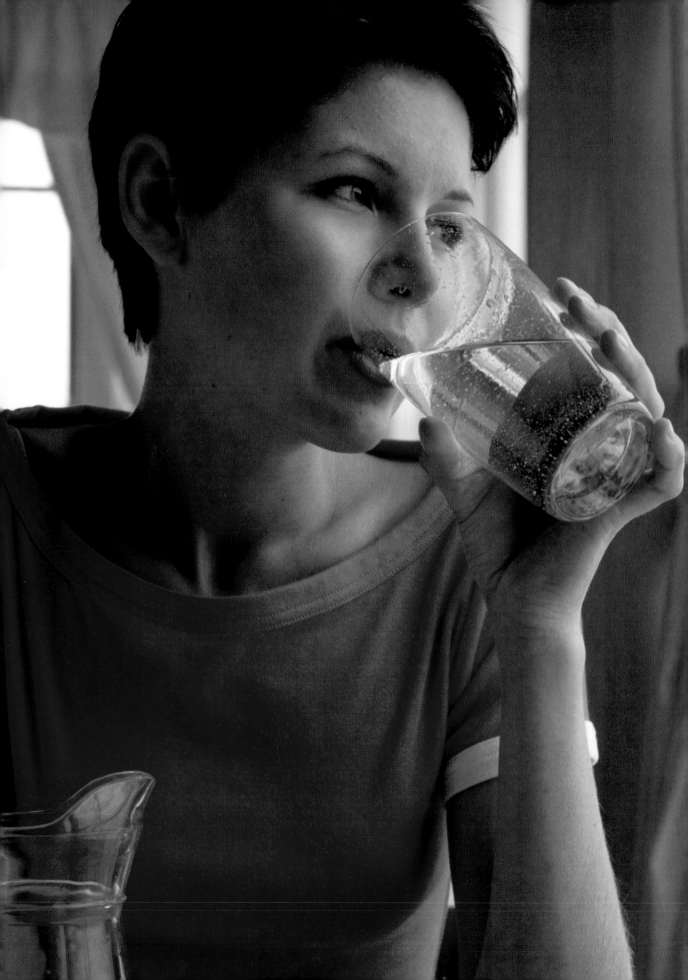

facing
the
future

By the time you finish the 28-Day Vitality Plan you should feel so much better that you will want to incorporate lots of elements from it into your everyday life. In fact, week four was a practice run for the rest of your life! It would be unrealistic, though, to imagine we can all keep to this level of diet, fitness and stress relief the whole time and so this brief chapter looks at how you can come back to the Plan in the future and utilize it at different ages and stages of your life.

the first day of the rest of your life

The Plan is over and you should be looking and feeling great – so now you need to think about which elements really benefited you during the past four weeks and how to incorporate them into your everyday routine. The first element to think about is diet. Because of the powerful detoxifying effect of this Plan – from the first week's juice fast right through to the nutritious meals in the last week – you are actually healthier on a cellular level. Your metabolism should be more finely tuned and the high levels of antioxidants in the Plan should have strengthened your immune system. So, before you rush for the fizzy drinks and the ready-made processed meals, think what an overload it would be on your now wonderfully cleansed system.

Juice it up

One of the easiest ways to keep up a high intake of anti-oxidants is to continue to drink one (or preferably two) fresh juices a day – one fruit and one vegetable is best. By now, you'll know how good these can taste and how filling they can be – without loading on worthless calories. If you run out of time, you can find some quite good substitutes on the supermarket shelves – orange, apple, carrot, usually – but make sure you're buying pure, fresh juices.

Your other really important liquid is water. Remember to drink at least 1.8 litres (3 pints) a day (some of it can be in herb teas, too) because this will continually flush everything through your digestive system and keep it cleansed. It also makes for easier elimination and prevents constipation (as do the juices).

Super food

Many of the meals in the Plan can easily be absorbed into daily life, though naturally you'll want to add others. Bear in mind a few simple guidelines for healthy eating:

- Eat plenty of fresh fruit and vegetables
- Avoid processed food and colourings, flavourings and preservatives whenever possible
- Avoid fizzy drinks – substitute juice or water
- Limit tea and coffee
- You can bring alcohol back into your diet, but bear in mind it is high in useless calories so limit yourself to drinking two or three times a week at most
- Bring meat back into your diet, too, if you like (you will have already brought back fish and chicken in the last week) but make sure it is lean and limit it to three times a week
- Above all, don't start smoking again!

Exercise

Try to keep to a regular exercise routine two to three times a week for cardiovascular fitness as well as bone density and muscle strength. Pick something you enjoy – you might like swimming, exercise classes, dance classes, cycling, trampolining – it doesn't really matter which you choose as long as you will stick to it over time. Best of all, mix several different forms of exercise – they will use different parts of the body.

Posture is something you can keep a check on as you go along – every now and again remember to correct the way you sit, walk or stand. If you walk well it will also help slim down your legs and shape your bottom – so it must be worth it!

You will know yourself if a particular part of your body needs toning – just choose the appropriate exercise. Make sure, though, that you aim for overall fitness rather than fixating on one single area.

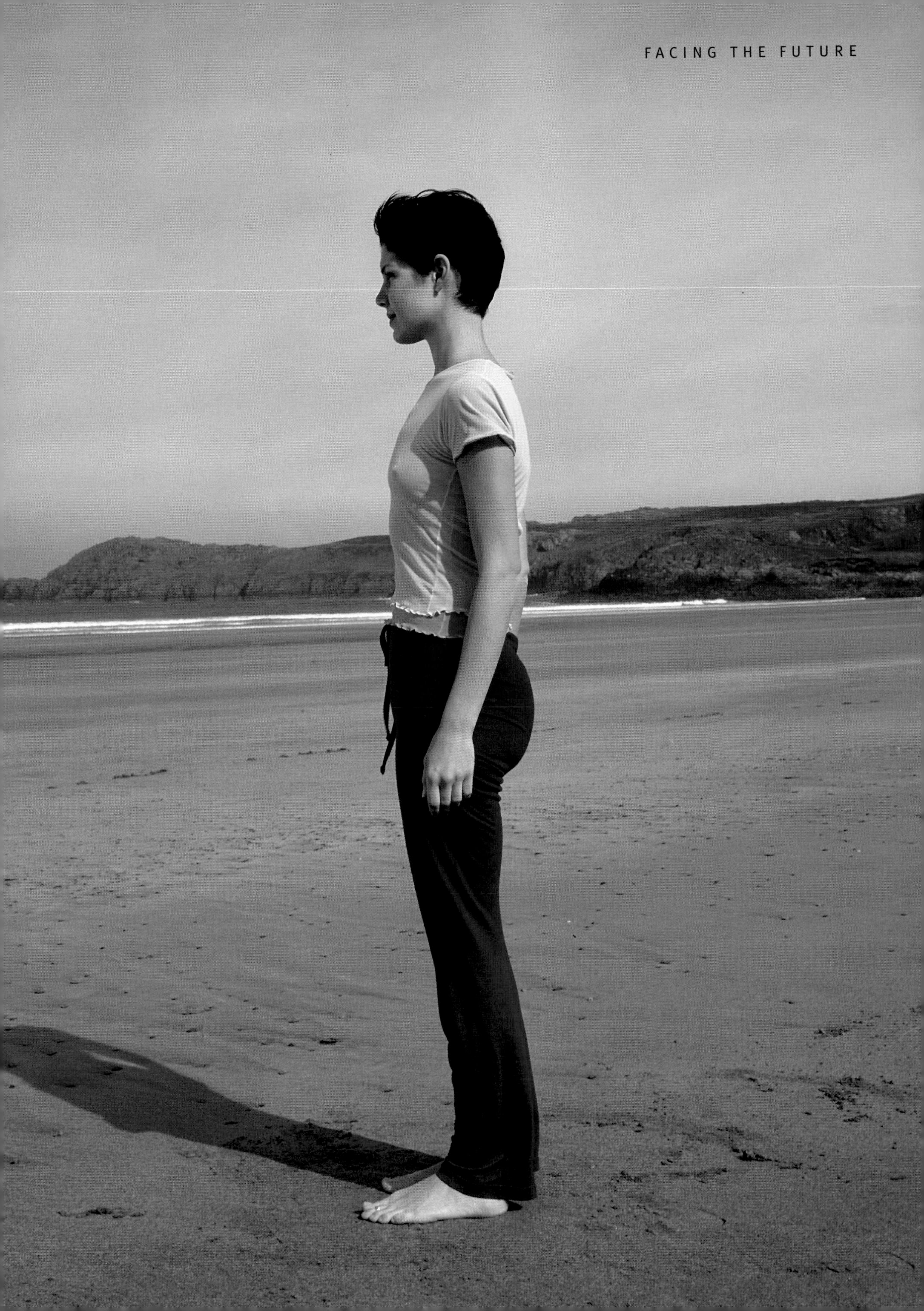

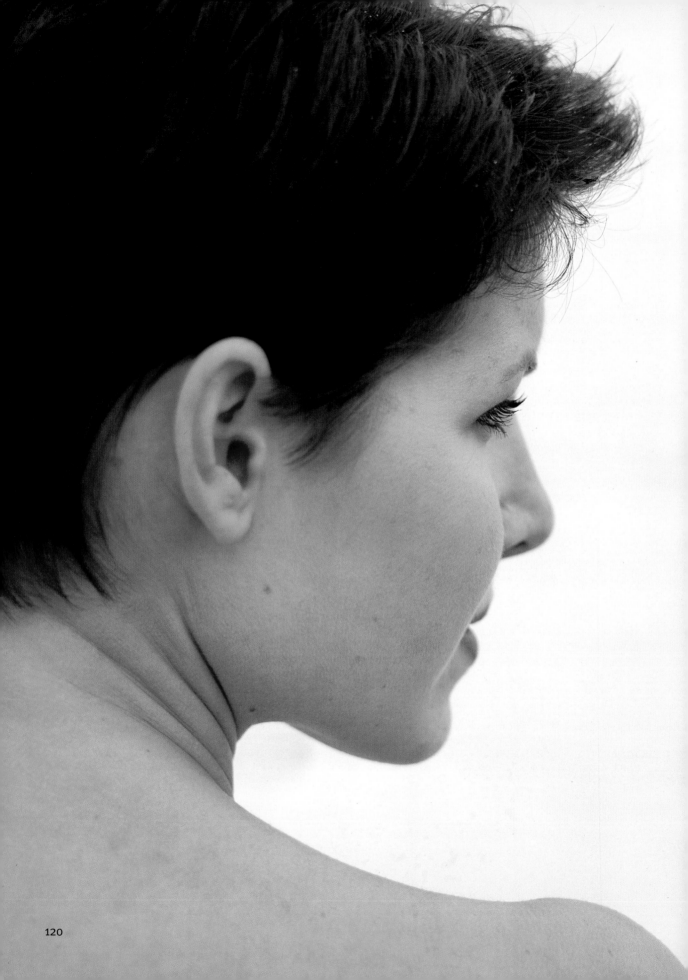

plan two

No matter how good their intentions may be, everyone falls by the wayside to some extent. We all know what Christmas, holidays, parties, birthdays and weddings bring with them – lots of over-indulgence – while moving home, changing jobs or undergoing partnership problems load on the stress. So, if you feel you need to be thoroughly detoxed, put on the right road again or simply given a spring clean, you can repeat the Plan again. It is advisable not to do it more than two or three times a year, though – just try modifying your diet and exercise routines the rest of the time.

If you began this Plan feeling very unfit or overweight, you may want to do it again to increase the impact. This is fine, but you should give yourself a six-week break before starting again, during which time you should keep to a sensible diet and exercise regime.

Ages and stages

As we all know, our bodies go through many different stages during the course of our lives. The Plan is not recommended for teenagers who are still growing, but by the end of the teens it can be very beneficial – particularly if, like many teenagers today, you have tended towards a rather inactive lifestyle, not to mention a craving for junk food!

During the course of a four-week plan, menstruation is pretty well inevitable at some point and it may be quite scanty compared to normal. Don't worry about this – it is quite a common reaction. If you suffer from menstrual cramps, try not to resort to painkillers as these will come as quite a shock to a cleansed system. Give yourself a gentle abdominal massage in a clockwise direction, using the following mixture:

Cramp Relief

5 drops chamomile essential oil
5 drops geranium essential oil
15 drops clary sage essential oil

Mix thoroughly in 50 ml (2 fl oz) of carrier oil.

You can also take clary sage oil internally for menstrual cramps and a combination of the two is very effective. Put 3 drops into a glass of water and mix thoroughly.

If you get headaches with your period, try massaging a few drops of lavender oil into your temples and on the back of your neck. Inhaling peppermint oil can be helpful if massage would be too painful. Finally, a bath with a few drops of peppermint, sweet marjoram or melissa can also be beneficial.

Motherhood

The 28-Day Vitality Plan is not recommended for anyone who is pregnant or breastfeeding. However, once you are past this stage, you will naturally want to get back in shape and you can do the Plan any time from four or five months after the birth – provided your general health is good. It is very important to check with your doctor before embarking on the Plan at any time, but especially if you have recently had a baby. You will need to take any exercises involving the abdominal muscles particularly gently – don't expect to be able to do any but the most basic of these exercises for some time. If you have had a baby in the last year, do no more than the waist twists and the most basic roll-ups in the Trim Torsos section. Take all stretches gently, too, and avoid any of the leg exercises where the legs are lifted and the abdominal muscles have to bear the weight.

Later life

Age is really no bar to the 28-Day Vitality Plan. If you are in good general health and would just like to improve on that, it is ideal. However, again you should check with your doctor, particularly if you have had any serious ailments or operations.

The main adaptation you will need to make is in terms of exercise. If you are very fit already there is no problem, but if you have not exercised regularly for some time, you should start very gently. Stick to walking and swimming for aerobic exercise, and in the body toning exercises only progress once you are comfortable with a set of exercises. The guidelines given in the week-by-week section are by no means to be strictly followed – everyone's body is different and it does not matter if you do not manage to do all the different exercises. What is important is that you exercise suitably for your own body, age and level of fitness.

progress charts

Fill in these pages to follow your progress as you go along. Some of your answers will be quite subjective – the quality of your skin and hair, for instance, will simply be how you regard your reflection in the mirror – while others, such as how you progress in the exercises, will be a clear measure of your achievement.

WEEK _____

Weight at start of week _____

Weight halfway through _____

DAY ONE

Food

What you had for:

Breakfast _____

Lunch _____

Dinner _____

Snacks _____

Drinks *(quantities)*

Juices _____

Broth _____

Herb teas _____

Water _____

Exercise

Fill in the exercises and time taken

Posture _____

Aerobic _____

Body toning _____

Techniques

Fill in how much time and your own estimation of effect

Skin brushing _____

Hydrotherapy _____

Baths _____

Relaxation _____

Meditation _____

Others _____

DAY TWO

Food

What you had for:

Breakfast _____

Lunch _____

Dinner _____

Snacks _____

Drinks *(quantities)*

Juices _____

Broth _____

Herb teas _____

Water _____

Exercise

Fill in the exercises and time taken

Posture _____

Aerobic _____

Body toning _____

Techniques

Fill in how much time and your own estimation of effect

Skin brushing _____

Hydrotherapy _____

Baths _____

Relaxation _____

Meditation _____

Others _____

DAY THREE

Food

What you had for:

Breakfast

Lunch

Dinner

Snacks

Drinks *(quantities)*

Juices

Broth

Herb teas

Water

Exercise

Fill in the exercises and time taken

Posture

Aerobic

Body toning

Techniques

Fill in how much time and your own estimation of effect

Skin brushing

Hydrotherapy

Baths

Relaxation

Meditation

Others

DAY FOUR

Food

What you had for:

Breakfast

Lunch

Dinner

Snacks

Drinks *(quantities)*

Juices

Broth

Herb teas

Water

Exercise

Fill in the exercises and time taken

Posture

Aerobic

Body toning

Techniques

Fill in how much time and your own estimation of effect

Skin brushing

Hydrotherapy

Baths

Relaxation

Meditation

Others

DAY FIVE

Food

What you had for:

Breakfast _____

Lunch _____

Dinner _____

Snacks _____

Drinks *(quantities)*

Juices _____

Broth _____

Herb teas _____

Water _____

Exercise

Fill in the exercises and time taken

Posture _____

Aerobic _____

Body toning _____

Techniques

Fill in how much time and your own estimation of effect

Skin brushing _____

Hydrotherapy _____

Baths _____

Relaxation _____

Meditation _____

Others _____

DAY SIX

Food

What you had for:

Breakfast _____

Lunch _____

Dinner _____

Snacks _____

Drinks *(quantities)*

Juices _____

Broth _____

Herb teas _____

Water _____

Exercise

Fill in the exercises and time taken

Posture _____

Aerobic _____

Body toning _____

Techniques

Fill in how much time and your own estimation of effect

Skin brushing _____

Hydrotherapy _____

Baths _____

Relaxation _____

Meditation _____

Others _____

height and weight charts

The weights below reflect frame as well as height for men and women (without clothes and in bare feet) aged 25 and over. Women aged 18–25 should deduct 450 g (1 lb) for each year below the age of 25.

DAY SEVEN

Food

What you had for:

Breakfast

Lunch

Dinner

Snacks

Drinks *(quantities)*

Juices

Broth

Herb teas

Water

Exercise

Fill in the exercises and time taken

Posture

Aerobic

Body toning

Techniques

Fill in how much time and your own estimation of effect

Skin brushing

Hydrotherapy

Baths

Relaxation

Meditation

Others

WOMEN

Height (cm/ft in)	Weight (kg/lb) Small frame	Medium frame	Large frame
142/4' 8"	41–44/90–96	43–48/94–105	46–53/102–117
145/4' 9"	42–45/92–99	44–49/96–108	47–54/104–120
147/4' 10"	43–46/94–102	45–50/99–111	49–56/107–123
150/4' 11"	44–48/97–105	46–52/102–114	50–57/110–126
152/5' 0"	45–49/100–108	47–53/105–117	51–59/113–129
155/5' 1"	47–50/103–111	49–54/108–120	53–60/116–132
157/5' 2"	48–52/106–114	50–56/111–124	54–62/119–136
160/5' 3"	49–53/109–117	52–58/114–128	56–64/123–140
163/5' 4"	51–55/112–121	54–60/118–133	58–65/127–144
165/5' 5"	53–57/116–125	55–62/122–137	59–67/131–148
168/5' 6"	54–58/120–129	57–64/126–141	61–69/135–152
170/5' 7"	56–60/124–133	59–66/130–145	63–71/139–156
173/5' 8"	58–63/128–138	61–68/134–149	65–73/143–161
175/5' 9"	60–64/132–142	63–69/138–153	67–75/147–166
178/5' 10"	62–66/136–146	64–71/142–157	68–78/151–171
180/5' 11"	64–68/141–151	67–73/147–162	71–80/156–176
183/6' 0"	66–71/146–156	69–76/152–167	73–83/161–183

MEN

Height (cm/ft in)	Weight (kg/lb) Small frame	Medium frame	Large frame
155/5' 1"	49–52/107–115	51–56/113–124	55–62/121–137
157/5' 2"	50–54/110–118	53–58/116–128	56–63/124–139
160/5' 3"	51–55/113–121	54–59/119–131	58–65/127–143
163/5' 4"	53–56/116–124	55–61/122–134	59–67/130–147
165/5' 5"	54–58/119–128	57–63/125–138	60–68/133–151
168/5' 6"	56–60/123–132	59–64/129–142	62–71/137–156
170/5' 7"	58–62/127–136	60–67/133–147	64–73/142–161
173/5' 8"	59–64/131–140	62–68/137–151	66–75/146–165
175/5' 9"	61–66/135–145	64–70/141–155	68–77/150–169
178/5' 10"	63–66/139–149	66–73/145–160	70–79/154–174
180/5' 11"	65–69/143–153	68–75/149–165	72–81/159–179
183/6' 0"	67–71/147–157	69–77/153–170	74–83/163–184
185/6' 1"	68–73/151–162	71–79/157–175	76–86/168–189
188/6' 2"	70–75/155–166	73–82/162–180	78–88/173–194
190/6' 3"	72–77/159–170	76–84/167–185	80–90/177–199

index

abhyanga massage 104–105
adrenalin 96
aerobic exercises 90, 109, 111, 112, 115
age 121
alcohol 9, 33
allergies 10
ankle trimmer 82
anti-oxidants 31, 32, 118
apple:
    gingered apples 46
    and grape juice 40
    juice 40, 43
    and pear juice 40
    and watermelon juice 40
arms 14
    crosses 86
    release 88
    stretches 63
aromatherapy:
    baths 95
    massage 104
artichoke juice 43
Ayurvedic health 104–105
Ayurvedic teas 38

baby corn with alfalfa 56
back 14
    stretch 21
beetroot juice 43
berries and apple juice 41
beta-endorphin 61
Bircher-Benner muesli 46
blackberry juice 43
body:
    renewal 30
    repair 32
    silhouette 9
    toning 109, 111, 112, 115
bosom firmer 86
bottom exercises 70–75
    back leg lifts 70
    buttock awareness 71
    deep pliés 75
    foot tapping 74
    leg circles 72
    leg stretches 72
    turn-out 74
breakfasts 46–47
    Bircher-Benner muesli 46
    gingered apples 46
    seedy yogurt 47
    stuffed figs 47
    yogurt fruit 47
breathing 13, 16
    exercises 6, 16
    meditations 101–102
bulgar wheat salad 53
buttocks 14
    awareness 71

cabbage juice 43
caffeine 9
cancer 31, 101
carrot:
    beetroot and cucumber juice 42
    juice 43
    parsley and cucumber juice 42
cat (exercise) 20
celeriac:
    onion and cucumber juice 42
    salad 55
celery juice 43
cells 30, 32
    renewal 31
centrifugal juicers 37
chamomile 38
cherry and grape juice 41
chicken tandoori 57
chickpea and watercress soup 51
child pose 89
Chinese noodles and prawns 59
chocolate 9
clenching fists 85
Cleopatra 95
coffee 9, 33
cold symptoms 35
continental mixed salad 55
cottage garden salad with strawberries 53
courgette and ginger soup 51
cranberry, apple and banana juice 41
crossed fists 69
cucumber juice 43
cycling 90

dancing 90
dandelion, carrot and turnip juice 42
Dead Sea mud 95
deep pliés 75
detox *see* detoxification
detoxification 6, 29, 30–31, 34
diet 6, 9, 29, 31, 111, 112, 115, 118
disease 29, 31, 96
double leg lifts 78–79
double leg stretch 82
drinks 38
drugs 33

elimination, excessive 34–35
elimination diet 10
essential oils 52, 95, 104
exercises 6, 9, 60–91, 118
    back stretch 21
    breathing 16
    cat 20
    plough 22
    roll down 14, 62, 65
    Salute to the Sun 24
    shoulder stand 22
    single leg stretch 19
    tennis ball 20

waist twist 18
    see also aerobic; bottom; head and shoulder; thigh; torso; warm-up; winding down

fasting, rules 33
fennel and cucumber juice 42
figs, stuffed 47
fish soup 51
flipper hands 86
flu symptoms 35
focusing 102
food:
    allergies 10
    intolerances 10
    raw 31, 32
foot tapping 74
free radicals 31, 96
French bean and apricot salad 55
fruit 31
    juices *see* fruit juices
    preparation 36
    soup, chilled 49
fruit juices 40–41
    apple 40
    apple and grape 40
    apple and pear 40
    apple and watermelon 40
    berries and apple 41
    cherry and grape 41
    cranberry, apple and banana 41
    melon 41
    pineapple, mango and papaya 41
    raspberry and peach 41
    rhubarb and apple 41
    tomato 41

ginger 38
Graham, Martha 18
Greek salad 54
guacamole and crudités 52

head 14
    rolls 84
head and shoulder exercises 84–87
    arm crosses 86
    bosom firmer 86
    clenching fists 85
    flipper hands 86
    head rolls 84
    shoulder lifts 84
headaches 34, 109, 121
heart disease 29, 31
herb tea 9, 38
hydraulic juice presses 37
hydrotherapy 94

illness 29, 31, 96
immune-boosting soup 50
immune system 94, 95, 96, 104

inner thigh lifts 77
irritability 34

jogging 90
Josephine 95
juice fast 6, 9, 10, 32, 34–35, 108
    breaking 35
    diet 35
    side-effects 34–35
juicers
    buying 37
    types 37
juices:
    fresh 6, 32, 118
    making 36–42
    recipes *see* fruit; remedial; vegetable juices
    ultimate detox 40

kidney (human) 32

lavender 95
legs 14
    circles 72
    kicks 81
    lifts 78
    stretches 72
    sweeps 80
lemon yogurt dressing 52
lentil soup 50
liver (human) 32
Louis XIV 95
lymphatic drainage 104

Maharishi Mahesh Yogi 99
main courses 56–59
    baby corn with alfalfa 56
    baked trout with dill and watercress 57
    chicken tandoori 57
    Chinese noodles and prawns 59
    grilled salmon and scallops 59
    hot scallop salad 57
    pasta with three herb sauce 58
    pasta with tomato sauce 58
    peperonata with noodles 58
    smoked trout and pasta 58
    steamed vegetables with ginger 56
    stir-fried vegetables 56
    vegetable hot-pot 56
mango juice 43
mantras 103
Mark Anthony 95
massage 104–105
meditation 98–103
    clinical research 101
    side-effects 101
    techniques 101–103
melon juice 41
menstruation 121

metabolism 30
minerals 48, 52, 95
mixed leaf salad with spiced nuts 55
Moor mud 95
motherhood 121
mud:
  Dead Sea 95
  Moor 95
muscle contrology 18
mushroom:
  courgette and tomato salad 52
  and mangetout soup 51

Napoleon 95
neck 14
neroli 95
noradrenalin 61, 96
nutrients 32

oils, essential 52, 95, 104

panchakarma 104–105
papaya juice 43
Paracelsus 95
parallel pliés 76
parsley:
  juice 43
  soup 50
parsnip:
  and carrot soup 48
  potato and celery juice 42
pasta:
  with three herb sauce 58
  with tomato sauce 58
peach juice 43
peperonata with noodles 58
pepper 48
peppermint 38
periods see menstruation
Pilates:
  Clara 18
  Joseph 18
  system 18
pineapple:
  juice 43
  mango and papaya juice 41

pliés 64
plough (exercise) 22
positive thinking 10
posture 6, 13–14, 108, 111, 112, 115
prawn, fennel and peach salad 54
pumpkin seeds 52
push me-pull yous 63

radicals see free radicals
raspberry:
  juice 43
  and peach juice 41
raw food 31, 32
recipes see breakfasts; juices; main
  courses; salad dressings; salads;
  soups

red leaf salad 53
relaxation 96–97
remedial juices 43
  apple 43
  artichoke 43
  beetroot 43
  blackberry 43
  cabbage 43
  carrot 43
  celery 43
  cucumber 43
  mango 43
  papaya 43
  parsley 43
  peach 43
  pineapple 43
  raspberry 43
  strawberry 43
  watercress 43
revitalizing stretch 88
rhubarb and apple juice 41
Robbins, Jerome 18
roll down 18
roll-ups 68
rope climbing (exercise) 69
rose oil 95
rosehip 38
rowing 90

salad dressings 52
  lemon yogurt 52
  sweet mustard 52
  tarragon and lemon 52
salads 52–55
  bulgar wheat 53
  celeriac 55
  continental mixed 55
  cottage garden with
    strawberries 53
  French bean and apricot 55
  Greek 54
  guacamole and crudités 52
  mixed leaf with spiced nuts 55
  mushroom, courgette and
    tomato 52
  prawn, fennel and peach 54
  red leaf 53
salmon and scallops 59
salt 48
Salute to the Sun 24
sandalwood oil 95
saunas 95
scallop salad, hot 57
scavengers 31
scissors (exercise) 69
selenium 31
sesame seeds 52
shallow breathing 16
shirodhara massage 105
shoulders 14
  circles 62
  lifts 84
  stand 22

shower routine 94–95
side stretches 66
single leg stretch 19
skin:
  brushing 94–95
  eruptions 35
skipping 90
smoking 9, 33
soups 48–51
  chickpea and watercress 51
  chilled fresh fruit 49
  chilled tomato 49
  courgette and ginger 51
  fish 51
  immune-boosting 50
  mushroom and mangetout 51
  parsley 50
  parsnip and carrot 48
  red lentil 50
  sweet potato 49
  vegetable stock 48
  yellow pepper 48
spinach, lettuce and carrot juice 42
spiritual meditation 103
St Denis, Ruth 18
stomach 14
strawberry juice 43
stress 16, 96
stretches 20–21
sunflower seeds 52
sweet mustard dressing 52
sweet potato soup 49
swimming 90

tarragon and lemon dressing 52
tea 9, 33
techniques 6, 93
tennis ball (exercise) 20
thigh exercises 76–83
  ankle trimmer 82
  double leg lifts 78–79
  double leg stretch 82
  inner thigh lifts 77
  leg kicks 81
  leg lifts 78
  leg sweeps 80
  parallel pliés 76
tiredness 35
tomato:
  juice 41
  soup, chilled 49
tongue, furry 34
torso exercises 66–69
  crossed fists 69
  roll-ups 68
  rope climbing 69
  scissors 69
  side stretches 66
  torso twists 66
  upper body circles 66
torso twists 66
toxins 31, 32, 34, 104
trampolining 90

transcendental mediation 99
treatments 93–95, 109, 111, 112, 115
triturating juicers 37
trout:
  with dill and watercress 57
  and pasta 58
turn-out 74

ultimate detox juice 40
upper body circles 66

vegetable:
  broth 38
  hot-pot 56
  juices see vegetable juices
  preparation 36
  stock 48
vegetable juices 42
  carrot, beetroot and cucumber 42
  carrot, parsley and cucumber 42
  celeriac, onion and cucumber 42
  dandelion, carrot and turnip 42
  fennel and cucumber 42
  parsnip, potato and celery 42
  spinach, lettuce and carrot 42
  watercress, carrot and celery 42
  white cabbage and cauliflower 42
vegetables 31
  stir-fried 56
  steamed with ginger 56
visualization 103
vitamins 9, 31, 48

waist twist 18
walking 90
warm-up exercises 62–65
  arm stretches 63
  pliés 64
  push me-pull yous 63
  shoulder circles 62
water 38, 94, 118
water treatments 94–95
watercress:
  carrot and celery juice 42
  juice 43
white cabbage and cauliflower
  juice 42
winding down exercises 88–89
  arm release 88
  child pose 89
  revitalizing stretch 88
World Health Organization 31

yellow pepper soup 48
yoga 24, 89
yogurt:
  seedy 47
  fruit 47

acknowledgements

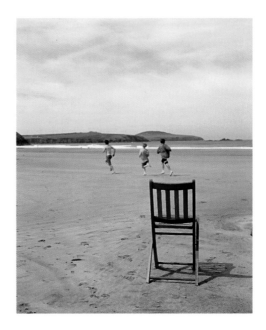

Published by Ulysses Press,
P.O. Box 3440
Berkeley, CA 94703-3440

ISBN 1-56975-190-0

Library of Congress Catalog Card
Number: 98-83028

Distributed in the United States by
Publishers Group West and in Canada
by Raincoast Books

First published in Great Britain in 1999
by Hamlyn, a division of Octopus
Publishing Group Limited

Printed in China

Model: Samantha Bilyk at Nevs agency

All special photography by Gary
Latham

Except for Octopus Publishing Group
Limited/Emma Peios 34 left, 38/
Graham Kirk 53, 54 right, 54 left, 57,
59 left, 59 right/Diana Miller 49, 50